Withdrawn

# THE STRESS EATING CURE

## LOSE WEIGHT with the NO-WILLPOWER SOLUTION to STRESS-HUNGER and CRAVINGS

**DR. RACHAEL F. HELLER, M.A., M.Ph., Ph.D.**
Assistant Clinical Professor Emeritus,
Mount Sinai School of Medicine, New York;
Assistant Professor Emeritus, Graduate Center of the City University
of New York, Department of Biomedical Sciences
and
**DR. RICHARD F. HELLER, M.S., Ph.D.**
Professor Emeritus, Mount Sinai School of Medicine, New York;
Professor Emeritus, Graduate Center of the City University
of New York, Department of Biomedical Sciences;
Professor Emeritus, Bronx Community College of the City University
of New York,
Department of Biology and Medical Laboratory Technology

RODALE

© 2010 by Rachael F. Heller, PhD, and Richard F. Heller, PhD

Rodale books may be purchased for business or promotional use or for special sales. For information, please write to:

Special Markets Department, Rodale Inc.,
733 Third Avenue, New York, NY 10017

Printed in the United States of America

Rodale Inc. makes every effort to use acid-free ♾, recycled paper ♻.

Book design by Chris Rhoads

**Library of Congress Cataloging-in-Publication Data**

Heller, Rachael F.
    The stress-eating cure : lose weight with the no-willpower solution to stress-hunger and cravings / Rachael F. Heller and Richard F. Heller.
        p.    cm.
    Includes index.
    ISBN-13 978–1–60529–456–8 hardcover
    ISBN-10 1–60529–456–X hardcover
    1. Weight loss.   2. Stress (Psychology)   3. Hunger.   4. Food habits.   I. Heller, Richard F.
II. Title.
    RM222.2.H362   2010
    613.2'5—dc22                                                                2010004830

Distributed to the trade by Macmillan

2   4   6   8   10   9   7   5   3   1   hardcover

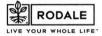

**We inspire and enable people to improve their lives and the world around them**

For more of our products visit **rodalestore.com** or call 800-848-4735

*This book is dedicated to our respected colleagues
in the scientific community.*

*Their insight, steadfast research, commitment, and hard work
have helped to make this discovery possible.*

# Contents

# PART IV

# PART V

# PART VI

# Stress-Eating Defined

The consumption of carbohydrate-rich and/or high-fat foods in response to mental, physical, or emotional stress.

Stress-eating is marked by a compelling hunger or by recurring, undeniable cravings that, *initially*, may be triggered by any of the following:

**overwhelming responsibilities**

**unrelenting demands**

**a sense of powerlessness**

**unexpressed anger or frustration**

**emotional abandonment**

**fear and/or worry**

**lack of sleep**

**boredom, loneliness, or disappointment**

**fatigue**

**anxiety**

**loss of a loved one**

**the need for a reward**

**many prescription and over-the-counter medications**

**an unpleasant, messy, or disorganized environment**

**excessive noise, heat, or cold**

Over time, an imbalance of hormones can trap the stress-eater in a Stress-Eating Cycle that is self-perpetuating when the initial stress trigger is no longer present.

The medical term for stress-eating is *stress-induced hyperphagia*, a condition that often goes undiagnosed and untreated.

Weight-loss diets do not address the physical cause of a stress-eater's cravings, hunger, and tendency to put weight on easily. It is little wonder that, in the long run, these diets are bound to fail.

*(continued)*

*The Stress-Eating Cure* is a program specifically designed to return the body to an optimal hormonal balance. Once the physical cause of stress-eating is eliminated, stress-hunger, cravings, stress-eating, and weight problems disappear—naturally.

A simple, Step-by-Step Plan as well as a Quick-Start Plan work to correct the *cause* of stress-eating and offer an end to the Stress-Eating Cycle—without struggle or sacrifice—for life.

# Acknowledgments

We wish to express our deep appreciation to:

Mel Berger, senior vice president, William Morris Agency. His remarkable insight and unique sense of humor never fail to amaze us. His thoughtful and incisive advice, exceptional mind, creativity, commitment, and thoughtful consideration make him the best literary agent in the world.

Shannon Welch, Rodale Inc., our extraordinary editor, for her intelligence, tireless work under pressure, unflagging interest, superb communication skills, and willingness to go the extra mile (time and time again) to get the job done (and done with excellence). Beyond all she does for so many every day, we thank her for her brilliant editing. Clearly, she has made this a far better book.

Hope Clarke, Rodale's remarkable senior project editor, for her steadfast attention to detail coupled with a rare ability to clarify and enhance the message. Her artistic abilities and commitment to excellence have made this book a perfect blend of the absolute best in form and function.

Graham C. Jaenicke, Mel Berger's most capable and intelligent assistant, for his trusted reliability, competence, professionalism, and unflagging involvement.

Charles Besford, general manager of Tokyo Disney Resort Hotels, and to his remarkable cast members. The wizard of the magnificent Tokyo Disneyland Hotel and his staff make our home away from home a joyful, healing, and most magical place.

Jacqueline Bik, MD, for her unswerving concern, staunch commitment, and the vast body of knowledge she brings to each patient's care.

Charles Davenport, MD, for his extraordinary expertise, constant competence, and remarkable compassion.

The outstanding staff at Partners Imaging of Sarasota, for their constant excellence, extraordinary sensitivity, and unswerving commitment to bringing the absolute best of care to their patients.

Philip Gutin, MD; Patsey Yeo-Ramakar, RN; and Beth Kurach, for the expertise, knowledge, compassion, and superb care they bring to so many who need it so greatly.

Rob Schloss and Chelsea Bauman, for their interest, daily input, critical advice, humor, and well-considered suggestions.

Apple Inc. and their support staff, for the development, care, and "feeding" of our user-friendly Macintosh laptops and desktops, which have made our lives wonderful. They have been invaluable tools in all of our work, as have Apple's excellent technical staff repair team, which keeps us up and running, and Apple's patient support staff, which regularly leads us out of the dark tech forest into the light. Apple's hard work and high standards have made our work both easy and productive. Because of Apple, we can say, we don't do windows.

# PART
# I

# Introduction

## *Stop the Blame. Correct the Cause.*

Stress-eaters don't give up easily. They may *want* to give up; they may wish they *would* give up; they may even tell themselves that they *are* giving up. But, sooner or later, something in them pushes them to try again to lose weight and get their eating under control.

If you are a stress-eater, chances are that you've subjected yourself to any number of diets of deprivation that demanded inordinate will-power and sacrifice. They limited your portion size, number of calories, or entire food groups. Certainly, when you restricted your intake or a type of food enough, you lost weight. For a time, each diet extracted its payment in hunger, exhaustion, irritability, and sleeplessness.

> *You can be deprived for only so long*
> *before you can't take it anymore.*
> *So, how can you blame yourself?*

Sooner or later, however, when you could no longer put up with the deprivation or when formerly forbidden foods were once again permitted (in impossibly tiny portions), you could hold back no longer.

Something may have triggered you. A loss, yet another demand, a great calamity, or a tiny incident. Whatever it was, it was enough to push you over the edge. You let go and ate what you had hungered for, for so long. After the damage had been done, you probably assumed you were at fault for not being able to stick with the diet. Rather than rightly blaming the diet for having made your life miserable, you wrongly blamed yourself!

Sound familiar? If so, good! Very good!

The greater the number of failed diets, the greater the likelihood that stress-eating has been your downfall. And that's good news because stress-eating is something we know how to handle.

3

*Insulin is only the tip of the iceberg.*
*To cure stress-eating, you must include*
*the latest in scientific discoveries.*

The program you'll find in the pages of this book has been designed to correct the hormonal imbalance that is the *cause* of cravings, stress-hunger,[1] and weight gain. There is a great deal more to stress-eating than insulin (the fat-regulating hormone). For decades, scientists have known that this hormone leads to cravings, hunger, and weight gain. Recently, however, researchers have discovered that insulin is but the tip of the iceberg.

In just the last few years, landmark scientific studies into the causes of stress-eating have revealed the power of two stress hormones, cortisol and its sidekick adrenaline, to summon four other hormones.

These four hormones, aptly termed the Masters of Metabolism, include ghrelin (the hunger hormone), serotonin (the satisfaction hormone), oxytocin (the hormone of affection, bonding, and sexuality), and leptin (the weight-loss regulator). These Masters of Metabolism, in combination with insulin, cortisol, and adrenaline, dictate how strongly you will crave food, how much you'll want to eat, how much weight you'll put on, and in what area of your body the fat will be deposited.

These hormones respond to your thoughts, feelings, and the world around you. In an attempt to help you deal with the stresses of daily life, they can send you virtually undeniable commands to seek out food and, after making it taste extraordinarily good, command your body to store that food energy away as fat.

Sheer willpower can hold these hormones at bay for only so long. Even as you deny yourself the food they make you crave, they will become more efficient at turning food energy into fat. So, even if you eat no more than you have in the past—or even less—you'll still gain weight. To make matters worse, they'll probably direct your body to store it around your middle.

---

[1] Stress-hunger is a compelling, sometimes overwhelming hunger based not on the body's need for food but on erroneous hormonal messages.

*You need only two things to beat stress-eating. You have them both!*

Working in harmony, these hormones might seem unbeatable. You may be tempted to conclude that you can't fight Mother Nature, and you'd be right, unless you could do one thing. To win back control of your eating, your weight, your health, and your life, you have to meet these hormones on their own grounds. No amount of willpower, positive thinking, or motivation is going to do it. If you want to win this battle, you're going to have to fight it as the *physical* disorder it is.

Your responsibility is to do just one thing: For the moment, allow in the possibility that, for all these years, your cravings, stress-hunger, and weight gain have been caused by a hormonal imbalance. Once you can acknowledge that your stress-eating may be the result of a *physical* disorder and, if so, must be *treated* as a physical disorder, you're halfway to being free of it for good.

The second thing you need in order to break free of stress-eating you hold in your hands. *The Stress-Eating Cure* has been specifically designed to correct the underlying hormonal imbalance that leads to stress-eating and the weight gain that follows.

*If you stress-eat, you have a physical disorder.*
*We know what causes it.*
*We know how to correct it—*
*without struggle, without sacrifice.*

The program you find within these pages will bring you the freedom to enjoy the foods you love every day without weighing or measuring portions or counting grams or calories. (Naturally slim people don't count, weigh, or measure; and, once your body is back in balance, you won't need to, either.) Best of all, as it eliminates the cause of your cravings and stress-hunger, this program will help shift your body into a fat-burning mode and help keep it there.

If you're ready to explore the possibility that you have a *physical* imbalance, you're about to discover all that you need—an effective and struggle-free cure for that imbalance—in the pages to come.

# 1

# Confessions

### RACHAEL'S CONFESSION:

The cravings were driving me crazy.

"I don't understand," I blurted out in frustration. "Why am I so hungry all of the time?"

It was the same question I had been repeating every day for months. I couldn't have expected my husband, Richard, to respond *yet again*, but when he didn't even look up from his work, I jumped at the chance for a showdown.

"Don't you even *care?*" I asked accusingly.

He looked up at me, his face expressionless.

"What?" I said, intent on provoking him. "Spit it out!"

As is his nature, he didn't rise to the bait.

"I was thinking," he answered with a quiet sadness.

"About what?" The nastiness in my voice had begun to fade, but only a little.

"I was just thinking that this should be the happiest time in our lives," he said simply.

*Everything I had fought for, throughout my life,*
*was about to slip through my fingers.*

The great knot in my stomach loosened and gave way to sobs. It was true. This was the moment I had been working for all of my life. I had everything I had ever dreamed of and so much more. Still, I wasn't happy. Even worse, I was on the brink of losing it all.

I had conquered the carbohydrate addiction that had ruled the first 38 years of my life. Once I had uncovered the insulin imbalance that was the cause of my cravings and discovered a simple way to correct it, I had been able to lose nearly 200 pounds and, more important, keep the weight off without a struggle.

For the last 15 years, I had looked and felt like a naturally slim woman. I had come to assume that I would always wear a size 6 petite and the overpowering hunger that had ruled my life in the past would never return.

Now, suddenly, it was about to slip away. Though I had not gone off the eating program that kept my carbohydrate addiction in check, something in me was different. Terribly different.

*An hour or two after I ate, I was back craving more.*

No matter how much I ate, no meal seemed to satisfy me. I was eating twice as much as I had in the past. The more I ate, the more it seemed that I wanted. Delicious meals that used to bring me satisfaction seemed to hold me for only a short time. Desserts only whetted my appetite for more.

Had I allowed myself, I could have snacked from morning 'til night.

*If I were to start bingeing again,*
*I knew I'd never stop.*

I was holding on to my self-control by a thread, and the thread was growing thinner and thinner. Though I looked the same to everyone else, I was one slip away from being more than 300 pounds again.

The terror in that thought brought my tears to a halt. I needed help. Real help. I needed my husband to really understand what was happening to me, how important it was, and how desperate I felt.

I forced myself to stay calm. Clearly, something was wrong with me. I suddenly heard the real meaning in my words. Though I'd been saying it all along, this time I really paid attention. My struggle was not simply the result of not trying hard enough or of not using enough willpower.

Something in my body was out of balance. The intense cravings; my powerful and recurring fantasies about food; my mood swings, foggy thinking, irritability, and anxiety; the feeling that I was not at peace in my mind or my body—all were coming from this imbalance, an imbalance that I knew had to have both a physical cause and a physical cure as well.

# RICHARD'S CONFESSION:

I love Rachael more than anyone can imagine, but she was driving me crazy! As she continued her relentless complaints about her cravings and hunger, I felt myself turn off and close up.

The truth was that I wasn't having such an easy time myself. Her fears were making me wonder if we were both about to go down the tube just when life couldn't have been sweeter.

*Oprah, Rosie, and* People *magazine!*
*Who could ask for more?*

We were about to appear on *Oprah* to talk about our highly successful treatment for carbohydrate addiction and our own personal successes as well. It was our third time back in 6 weeks, and once again, we were to be her exclusive guests. On Amazon.com, we held the top eight spots in the world, with more than five million of our books in print. We vacationed with Rosie O'Donnell, Demi Moore, and many other of this country's biggest celebrities, and *People* magazine was about to feature us in their upcoming issue. It felt as if there were no stopping us.

*I was hoping Rachael's cravings would just disappear.*
*I was not about to tell her that I was getting them, too.*

The only thing that threatened to spoil it all was Rachael's continuing complaints—and the fear they stirred way down deep inside me. A fear I was fighting hard to deny.

# 2

# Confrontations

## RACHAEL:

If you've ever seen one of those cartoons in which a little dog sinks his teeth into someone's leg and won't let go, you have a pretty accurate view of me at my best (and most trying). I am tenacious, persistent to a fault. I hate to think I didn't give something my best. I don't give up easily, and, most certainly, I don't give up without a fight.

Once I pitted myself against the problem that was *causing* my cravings and hunger (instead of blaming myself for them), I found myself in familiar territory. I had conquered this type of problem before. Against all odds. And I had done it alone.

Now, with Richard at my side, I thought it would be far easier. I was in for a big surprise.

> *Going it alone had been rough.*
> *Solving the problem with help, however,*
> *was about to prove far more difficult.*

Years earlier, when I had discovered the cause of my addiction to carbohydrates, I hadn't cared what anyone thought about my ideas, and I gave myself full rein to consider every possibility. I answered to no one for my time, energy, productivity, or thinking. In the end, that freedom allowed me to learn all that I needed to learn, to test and retest my hypotheses, and, finally, to succeed.

Now, facing a new problem, I was in a different situation. My time was no longer my own. I was already torn between doing research and teaching with Richard at Mount Sinai School of Medicine in New York, authoring our 9th and 10th books, and more television, radio, and print interviews than I could possibly keep track of.

Each day, we were being bombarded with hundreds of phone calls, e-mails, and letters from people who desperately needed help. Yet, my own cravings and hunger had become so intense that I could barely think.

*Everything I ate and drank had suddenly
become everyone else's business.*

With this newly won fame, my eating and my weight were under constant scrutiny by what seemed to be the entire world. I could not eat a meal at a restaurant without at least one person commenting on the fact that, indeed, I did eat just as I had recommended in our books. I couldn't eat in the company of friends or family without fielding comments and questions about everything on my plate.

On one occasion, a neighbor took the glass from my hand and took a sip of my drink to confirm that, indeed, I was drinking unsweetened iced tea!

"You've got to be very strict with yourself," she said sternly. "You've got a lot of people who consider you their role model!"

While I had no intention of going off my eating program, knowing that so many people were watching and questioning everything I put in my mouth almost made me feel like rebelling.

*I had lost nearly 200 pounds,
but, to me, in every video and photo,
I still looked fat.*

The pressure of television appearances and publicity photos added an overwhelming responsibility for me to be ever watchful of my weight. I became extraordinarily critical (even more than I had been) of every aspect of my appearance.

I remember thinking that, not so many years earlier, I had been imprisoned in a 320-pound body that everyone stared at and judged me for. Now, though I was a size 6 petite, I was still being stared at and judged. It felt as if nothing I would ever do would be good enough, and, at every moment, I was on the brink of failing.

With these thoughts in my mind and that terror in my heart, my cravings and desire to once again start bingeing became unbearable. I was barely holding it together. Then a simple comment threatened to push me over the edge.

*One casual comment brought me*
*to the brink of disaster.*

I was visiting the City University of New York Graduate Center, where I had earned my doctorate many years earlier. I chanced upon Jim, the security guard who had greeted me almost every morning during my 8-year tenure at the school. He had known me in my formerly fat state, and in the last years before I graduated, he had watched me take off the pounds as well.

On the day of my visit, his smile was as warm as ever, and he welcomed me as he had every day when I had been a student. Suddenly, he stopped, shook his head, took a step back, and revealed what had really been going through his mind during the many years of our acquaintance.

"You know," he said, "I've got to tell you how great you look now. I mean, compared with what you used to look like."

I was shocked and uncertain how to respond.

"It's really something," he continued. "I mean you were fat. Really fat. And not just pleasantly plump fat but, you know, sloppy fat. . . . "

He nodded confirmation, apparently reveling in the memory.

In no uncertain terms, Jim went on to explain that, when he had first seen me, he could not believe that the university would admit someone who looked like me into the psychology program.

"I mean, you looked like your own mother," he added. "Or grandmother," he chuckled. "I mean to tell you, you were really fat."

At that point, he raised his hands to his sides to indicate the wide girth of my former self.

I stood speechless. Obviously, this man, one whom I had smiled at and greeted on countless occasions, one for whom I had a distant fondness, thought he was complimenting me.

"Doesn't he *hear* what he is *saying?*" I thought disbelievingly.

I saw myself through his eyes. I was filled with shame.

I opened my mouth, though I'm not certain what I was going to say, when a few, final words from Jim stopped any thought of response.

"And, lookey here!" he continued with a broad grin. Unexpectedly, he had taken my hand and was almost spinning me around. "You still haven't gained it back. No, siree! Not yet!"

> *His casual comment unleashed the terror*
> *I had been fighting hard to hold back.*

That was it: my breaking point, the moment I had been dreading, when all the feelings I had been struggling to keep under control broke free. In those few words and all they implied lay my terrors, past, present, and future.

It was just as I always feared. The people I had thought of as friends were watching me, waiting for my inevitable failure. Though they never let on, each was certain that, sooner or later, I would once again become the hideous monster they could almost enjoy being repulsed by. In that moment, I saw myself through their eyes: gluttonous, self-destructive, weak-willed, and piggish. It was horrifying, but I knew it was true.

I could barely catch my breath. My heart beat so frantically I could barely stand it. All of the pressure, demands, expectations, and fear that I would fail came tumbling down in an avalanche of anxiety.

I muttered something about not feeling well, which, from my pallor, Jim apparently believed to be true. I turned and walked out of the building, never making my way to the meeting that had brought me there that fateful morning.

Instead, I retreated to the coffee shop across the street from the Graduate Center. It was a familiar place of comfort, one in which I had binged my way through my first year of graduate studies and where, in the years that followed, I was able to get the food that would satisfy me and sustain me on my weight-loss program.

I cringed at the thought of meeting old acquaintances, especially the manager and his waitresses, who had cheered me along. "God knows what they really thought," I said to myself.

I settled into a corner table, grateful that, on that day, all the faces at the coffee shop were unfamiliar. There, with a plain tea and lemon before me, still reeling from the awareness of what countless acquaintances and friends had really thought of me, a miracle happened.

# 3

# Connections

## RACHAEL:

For me, it was a miracle. Truly. In that instant, something in me changed. Profoundly.

It took a moment to figure out what was different. Something was missing, and it felt wonderful!

> *Suddenly, the cravings were gone.*
> *The hunger had vanished.*

For the first time in as long as I could remember, my mind was quiet; no voices were calling me names or predicting dire consequences for my every thought or action. Even more than that, there was a stillness in my mind and body . . . like the calm after a battle has suddenly ceased.

That was it! There was no struggle. For the first time in months, maybe years, my body wasn't steeled against my need to satisfy my hunger. My body and my mind were no longer at war.

And I knew why. After seeing myself through Jim's eyes, I had hit rock bottom. I had realized that no matter how hard I tried, I could never make people understand what it was like to fight endless battles with food and weight, to bear the memory of a thousand cruel remarks, or to be trapped in a body that had been disfigured by the gain and loss of hundreds of pounds. Most of all, I would never be able to convince those who did not want to know that a *physical* imbalance had been the cause.

Then a second and far more important truth became clear. In trying so hard to be the living proof that an addiction to carbohydrates had a physical cause, I had set off a far more powerful physical imbalance in my own body!

A deep peace washed over me. It was the same peace I had known for years following my discovery of my addiction to carbohydrates. I had the answer I had been begging Richard to give me but which we both knew I would have to discover myself.

*Carbohydrate addiction had been only the tip of the iceberg.*
*The waters had receded now, and*
*a whole new problem had revealed itself.*

The reason why my cravings and hunger had returned was not related to a recurring addiction to carbohydrates but, rather, to a far deeper problem. It was a problem that had been buried beneath my addiction to carbohydrates and had not surfaced until now.

Just as a person who is allergic to strawberries may never know there is a problem until he or she eats the first berry, so this second problem, whatever it was, had not emerged until something in the environment activated it.

That "something" was not hard to pinpoint. Only moments earlier, I had given myself permission to give up, to stop fighting. With those thoughts, the stress that I had been living with for so long slipped away. As the stress disappeared, so did the hunger and cravings. It was a connection that was well known and well documented. Scientists had been writing about it for decades; Richard and I had touched on it in our own writings. Still, I had never taken it in and applied it to my own cravings, hunger, and weight gain.

Perhaps the problem was that stress-eating has become so commonplace, it's almost taken for granted. It's been portrayed in a hundred sitcoms and movies. But for me and, perhaps, for countless others, it was no laughing matter.

What to do about it? That was a whole different problem.

Until that day, I held firmly to the belief that stress-eating was something you could manage if you just tried hard enough, if you just used a little willpower.

When the topic had come up in our research groups, I had offered some commonplace suggestions. In truth, I hadn't given the problem very much consideration because I had failed to recognize the true power of stress.

All these years, I had never considered exploring the problem of stress-eating as I would any other physical problem.

*There was work to be done.*
*For myself and for others.*
*I was home again!*

I decided that Richard and I had to start work immediately on the cause of and treatment for stress-eating. We'd write up a new research protocol for the medical center, begin gathering data, and once the current media interviews were concluded, we would . . . My mind jumped back onto the same old treadmill and, in an instant, the hunger and cravings were back. With a vengeance.

I sat stock-still and, for a moment, seriously considered eating anything I could get my hands on in order to satisfy the newest burst of cravings.

But the fighter in me kicked in, and the thrill of the hunt, the chance to solve a new problem—for myself and for others—was more tempting than any food I could imagine.

I did the only sane thing possible. I called for help.

*That's when Richard stepped in and,*
*I firmly believe, saved my life.*

# RICHARD:

When Rachael phoned me from New York, she didn't mince words.

"I know what's going on!" she began. "These cravings and hunger are coming from some physical problem, some imbalance or something. I know it's all related to stress in some way, but I don't know how."

She went on to explain that we were going to have to make time in our impossibly overburdened schedule to figure out what was happening to her and to find a treatment.

I agreed, though I had no idea how we might fit more work time into our day unless we did away with sleep altogether. So, essentially, I humored her and said, "Sure, we'll check it out." Then I said good-bye, quite pleased with my "yes, dear" approach to her call for help.

Something in me would not let me put the matter to rest, however. It was just this voice that kept repeating one simple thought and, with it, made me see past all of the less-important things that had taken over my life.

*If she truly had some kind of illness,*
*I'd put everything on hold and help her.*
*Why would I do any less when it comes to this?*

"If Rachael *really* had a physical problem, as she says she does," the voice insisted, "what would you do?"

The answer was simple. I would drop everything and do whatever needed to be done to help her. Why then, I asked myself, wasn't I doing that now?

Within days, I stopped, simply stopped, everything that had been driving the machine of our lives. I put our research on hold, assigned our medical students appropriate independent study projects, called a halt to all media appearances, and told family and friends we were incommunicado.

"For how long?" they asked.

"For as long as it takes," I replied.

# 4

# The Cure

## RACHAEL AND RICHARD:

In some ways, it was the most courageous thing we had ever done. Alone in our home together, no phone, no e-mail, no friends or family, no distractions. Just us and the problem we were committed to solving. And thousands of pages of notes from our years of research.

*We had become "urban hermits."*

Closing ourselves off from the world felt as if we had been banished to our room and told that we couldn't come out until we had accomplished a seemingly impossible task. We had become "urban hermits," isolated in one of the most crowded cities in the world.

Still, we held on to the belief that the only way to get to the other side of a problem was by going through it, head-on, and we promised ourselves that the freedom that lay on the other side would be that much sweeter for all the sacrifice.

And sweet it was. In less than a month, we had the answer. Or, at least what we hoped would be one of the answers.

Together, we had analyzed every strategy that had helped stop stress-eating in our research subjects at the medical center. Some strategies had been of our own creation, based on a combination of intuition, experience, and knowledge of the physical effects of stress on the body. Other tactics, however, came from our research subjects or from readers who had sent us countless e-mails and letters, thanking us and updating us on their progress.

*Every flat surface in our home—chairs, desks, even the floors*—
*was covered with stacks of books and piles of notes.*

Of all the successes we reviewed, we carefully chose only those stress-eating reduction techniques that met two criteria: They had to prove repeatedly to break the Stress-Eating Cycle, and, at the same time, they had to require very little effort or time.

Knowing *what* works, however, is of little value to the scientist, who must also have an explanation *why* the indicated treatment works.

That's where we were running into difficulty. When we searched for an explanation, a physical change that would explain why these strategies had helped break the cycle of stress-eating, each strategy seemed to be tied to any one of six or seven different hormonal imbalances.

*As long as we were focused on the villain,*
*we would never succeed.*

In the past, we had identified insulin as the culprit in carbohydrate addiction. Strategies that helped reduce the cravings, hunger, weight gain, and blood sugar swings associated with carbohydrate addiction worked because they helped to balance insulin levels in the body. When it came to stress-eating, however, we simply could not pinpoint the one hormonal imbalance that was causing it.

The answer, of course, was right there in front of our eyes, and if we hadn't been so fixed on the idea of a single answer, we probably could have saved ourselves a lot of work.

In the end, stress, itself, revealed the answer. As the weeks passed, we began to notice changes in our personalities, our interactions with each other, and our abilities to concentrate. With each change, there were corresponding increases in our cravings and hunger.

A sudden decrease in desire for personal contact was associated with an intense craving for sweets (which were most enjoyed when eaten in private). An increased desire for conversation was accompanied by a hunger for spicy foods. A very warm bath decreased cravings and hunger and, at the same time, reduced all interest in task-related responsibilities.

*Our bodies were being taken over*
*by a gang of powerful hormones.*
*One after another, each was taking control.*

When we considered the fact that the changes that were taking over our bodies were not the result of a single hormonal process, the reason why we could find no single, effective treatment for stress-eating became obvious! Stress-eating was the result of several *different* hormonal imbalances that moved through the stress-eater's body in chemical waves of rapid succession.

At any moment, one hormone might reign supreme over all the others, only to be replaced, in a matter of seconds, by another. No single hormone acts alone, so with each new fluctuation, the body was being thrown into yet another state of imbalance.

It took more than an additional year of research, examination, and reexamination to tease out the major players in this war of hormones and map the battlefield. In the end, however, the pieces came together like a great jigsaw puzzle. The more we discovered, the more the bigger picture made sense.

Then came the hard part. Each hypothesis, each piece of the puzzle that explained the hormonal web of stress-eating, needed to be tested. If we were right, the strategies and tactics would bring indisputable relief from the cravings and hunger and, in a short time, would lead to struggle-free weight loss.

We had designed the program to correct the hormonal imbalances we believed were the cause of stress-eating. If we were right, we'd know it soon. And if we weren't, we were about to find that out as well.

*We called on a decade of faithful research subjects whom we*
*had helped in the past. Now, we needed their help.*

We put out a call to our research subjects, old and new. We invited them to take part in an eating experiment that we believed would bring them the weight loss and the freedom from hunger and cravings that they were seeking.

We detailed the program (which today has become the Quick-Start Plan of *The Stress-Eating Cure* that you will find in the pages that follow). We told them to first get the okay from their private physicians, and then we sat back, held our collective breath, and waited.

*We didn't have to wait long for the verdict.*

Within a week, we had our first answer. Margaret, one of our newest research subjects, was on the phone. Her voice was so loud with excitement that we had to hold the receiver away from our ears.

"I can't believe it," she shouted. "It's the most amazing thing I've ever experienced! All I did was change a few simple things, and, just like that, the cravings are gone."

Margaret's voice grew softer and more hesitant as she continued. "It doesn't make sense. Maybe I'm just wanting it to work," she said thoughtfully. "Maybe I just want the cravings to be gone so much that I'm convincing myself this is going to make all the difference."

We heard the longing in Margaret's voice, and we wanted to reassure her. But, more than anything, we knew that it would be an injustice to her to offer her false promises.

We agreed it was possible that she was experiencing a placebo effect. Still, she had never experienced that kind of reaction in the past.

"We'll just have to wait and see. Keep doing what you're doing," we concluded.

"Keep doing what I'm doing," Margaret said with a laugh. "Nothing could make me change a thing!"

*The good news might have been nothing*
*but a placebo effect. Only time would tell.*

The second and third calls followed within a day, and over the next few days, nearly a quarter of our research subjects had called to report the same remarkable results.

The rest of the week followed suit. It had become obvious—even to our scrupulously cautious way of thinking—that we had succeeded.

The work was far from over, we told each other. In fact, it had just begun. Testing, retesting, refining the program, adding a tested Step-by-Step Plan (which you will also find in the pages that follow), and anticipating all of the challenges, needs, and preferences that stress-eaters might experience would require a great deal of work.

*It took twice as long as we estimated.*
*And brought us a hundred times the happiness.*

We estimated the final touches on our cure for stress-eating would take about 3 years, 5 at the most. In the end, it took almost twice that time: a decade of work.

It was a big chunk of our lives; but, thinking back on all of the joyous faces, the healthier and happier lives this program has made possible, and our own hard-won and dearly treasured freedom from cravings, hunger, stress-eating, and weight gain, it has been more, far more, than worth it!

# TODAY

Today, we are healthy, happy, and slim. We've lost a combined weight of more than 250 pounds, and we've kept it off for more than 25 years. Most important, we've remained slim and healthy without sacrifice or struggle.

We handle the stresses of daily life, work, and family without even the thought of turning to food for comfort or reward (though every day we enjoy the food we love).

We don't need to use willpower or muster one bit of determination. We've corrected the physical cause of our stress-eating and weight gain, and, best of all, we live without the fear of ever gaining it back.

# PART
## II

# 5

# Stress *Can* Make You Fat!

Today, stress-eating seems to be on everyone's mind. A quick search on Google reveals more than 10 million sites devoted to the topic. Thousands of news articles herald warnings that stress-eating has taken this country by storm.

"Is Stress Making You Fat?"
   —ABC News, March 20, 2009

"When Economy Sours, Tootsie Rolls Soothe Souls"
   —*The New York Times*, March 23, 2009

"When Times Get Tough, the Tough Crave Candy"
   —*El Paso Times*, March 29, 2009

"Plunging Dow, Soaring Scales: Beware of 'Recession Obesity'"
   —*USA Today*, March 8, 2009

"Recession Has a Sweet Side: When the Going Gets Tough, the Tough Get Chocolate"
   —*Hamilton Spectator*, March 27, 2009

"Do You Have a Stress-Induced Sweet Tooth?"
   —*Self* magazine, March 24, 2009

"Is Daily Stress Making Us Fat?"
   —Courier-Journal.com, March 12, 2009

"Candy Takes the Bite Out of Tough Times: Adults Turning
to Candy to Beat the Stress of Recession"
—*Star Telegram*, March 29, 2009

"Candy Sales Sweeten Recession Woes"
—NBC News, March 24, 2009

For virtually every American, these headlines confirm a truth we already know only too well: The ups and downs of a volatile economy and the overwhelming demands of daily life are taking their toll.

# TRIPLE PLAY

The too-often-repeated, old-world description of stress has little relevance to what most of us experience as stress every day. For decades, authorities have explained that when your body senses a challenge to your well-being, your hormones rally to protect you. In prehistoric times, this "fight-or-flight response" was meant to defend you against threats from predators or aggressors.

While all of this is true, it does not explain why, in modern times, we experience stress when faced with challenges that, clearly, are *not* a matter of life and death.

*In today's world, stress might be best imagined
as a three-way tug-of-war between our
minds, bodies, and emotions.*

When it comes to our minds, bodies, and emotions, we may find ourselves pulled in three directions at once. Our minds evaluate a situation, recall past experiences, make judgments, and arrive at decisions. Our bodies react to a whole host of hormonal fluctuations and urge us to do whatever is needed to keep those hormones in balance. Our emotions reflect our desires, hopes, and fears. Each of these—mind, body, and emotions—influences the other two. Under the best of circumstances, they work together to keep us safe and well and to make us happy.

*When feelings and actions match, no stress.*
*When feelings and actions don't match, lots of stress.*

What happens when one of these three factions is at odds with the others? The answer is simple. We feel stressed. Even if we don't recognize it as stress, we find ourselves irritable, out-of-sorts, negative, blue, emotional, nervous, or the like. We may know that we are overreacting to situations but find that we are helpless or have no desire to change our response. Motivation, enthusiasm, and joy all disappear. This is stress in action. And it takes over our minds, bodies, and emotions when one part of us strongly wants to do something and another cannot or will not. This conflict may occur when we are confronted with an unpleasant situation or when we encounter what others might consider a pleasant experience as well.

*Tell someone what you really feel,*
*and the stress disappears.*
*Feel guilty about what you just did,*
*and the stress returns.*

Imagine, for a moment, that there is someone to whom you wish you could reveal the negative feelings that you have been hiding. Let's say that, in fact, you speak honestly, expressing all that you've been feeling.

Chances are, at least for a moment, you will no longer feel stressed. In fact, you might be surprised at the feeling of freedom that you experience. Your mind has given you the okay to do what your emotions have been longing for and your body has been aching to do. There is no stress because there is no tug-of-war.

On the other hand, reconsider the same scenario in which you want to express those same negative feelings. This time, however, imagine that you hold your tongue. Most likely, you experience the typical symptoms of stress: Your stomach tightens, your heart beats faster, and your muscles tense. Your mind has stopped you from doing the very thing that your emotions and body most desire. And, in a rush of hormones, your emotions and body are sending you the message that they are not happy!

*If you experience stress when you're happy,*
*you might not be so happy after all.*

Why, then, do we sometimes stress-eat when we're happy? The answer is the same! Though one part of us, our mind, for example, may tell us that a situation is good and that we *should* be happy, our feelings may reveal a different reality.

Let's say that, as an anniversary celebration, your husband surprises you with a lovely dinner at your favorite restaurant. You should be pleased, you tell yourself, and you categorize this as a happy occasion. Why, you wonder, even as you are getting dressed, even though you aren't all that terribly hungry, are you reaching for candy by the handful?

The answer is that, perhaps, you aren't all that pleased. Not really. With a moment to consider how you *really* feel, you might discover that you have no desire to go out to eat at that time. You have just come home from work and you are tired; you have an important task at home that you wanted to complete that evening (assuming you could keep your eyes open); and, the truth is, you know your husband came up with the restaurant celebration at the last minute because he hadn't taken the time, forethought, or energy that would have been required to get you a gift that you might really have wanted.

Though you might wish you felt otherwise, down deep you know that this is *not* a happy occasion. The fact that you are grabbing handfuls of candy even as you are getting ready to go out to eat—especially when you aren't all that hungry—is a clear sign of stress-eating. Your attempt to stress-eat the feelings away reveals that at least one part of you is not willing to pretend that all is just fine.

Guilt, distrust, or resentment (though well-founded) can, in the same way, put you at odds with what others might consider to be a very pleasant experience. It's not a happy occasion if *you* don't *feel* happy.

Feeling stressed at a time that normally would be considered a happy occasion does not *always* reveal a conflict between feelings and thoughts, however. Though you may not be aware of the fact, your body may be fighting a battle of its own.

*Some of the foods you least suspect can
easily trigger a full-blown stress reaction.
But you don't have to give them up.*

There are times when your body is in the throes of a hormonal imbalance as a result of the kind of food you've been eating or the frequency with which you've been eating it.

Sugary foods are a prime example, though other foods can trigger hormonal imbalances as well. Most of us know the power that sugar has to bring us pleasure and relieve some of the stresses of the day. The pleasure disappears quickly, however, and a short time after eating sugary treats, you may find yourself in an emotional free fall.

Your heart may start pounding. You may feel sweaty, light-headed, headachy, or irritable. You may crave more . . . and more. Why? Your hormonal balance has fallen into chaos. Your body is in the throes of a full-fledged stress reaction.

Though, in this instance, your mind and feelings were *not* at odds with each other, a great hormonal storm is taking place within you. Whether or not you experience it as such, this hormonal imbalance is experienced by the body as significantly stressful.

*The very thing that makes you stress-eat can set you free—
without giving up the foods you love most!*

Depending on your body's genetic makeup, a wide variety of foods may throw your body's hormonal balance out of kilter. There is no way to avoid all of these trigger foods. Besides, past diet defeats have shown you that giving up the food you love most simply doesn't work.

The solution, the cure, is simple. It comes from discovering what makes your body different from the body of a non-stress-eater, then *using* that knowledge to stop stress-eating in its tracks.

# 6

# Eaters Are from Mars, Stress-Eaters Are from Venus

Why do some people turn to food when they are tired . . . or sad . . . or worried . . . or angry (or all of the above)? Why is it that others do not? When faced with a stressful situation, what causes some people to feel as if they *have* to eat and others to lose their appetite? Why do some people eat *after* the stress has passed? The answer to all of these questions lies in the fact that not all eaters are created equal.

*Some of us are born Stress-Resisters. Some are born Stress-Responders. But you can change what nature gave you.*

## STRESS-RESISTERS

To understand why some people become stress-eaters and others do not, one simply has to understand the difference between Stress-Resisters and Stress-Responders.

*Stress-Resisters are not likely to become stress-eaters.*

If you were a Stress-Resister, chances are you would not become a stress-eater. Stress-Resisters have bodies that, by their physical nature, are able to modulate the normal stress response. When a person is faced with stress, a tiny region at the base of the brain sets off an alarm system in the body. Through a combination of nerve and hormonal signals, this system prompts the adrenal glands, located atop the kidneys, to release a surge of hormones, including adrenaline and cortisol.

Adrenaline increases the heart rate and raises blood pressure. Cortisol, the primary stress hormone, increases sugars (glucose) in the bloodstream and makes the sugar more available to the brain. Cortisol also curbs nonessential functions (including digestion, reproduction, and the growth process) so that the body can focus all of its energies on the more immediate challenge.

Stress-Resisters seem to produce just the right amount of hormones for thriving in today's world. When, in the face of stress, cortisol temporarily puts nonessential functions on hold, Stress-Resisters simply do not feel like eating or having sex.

When the threat has passed and the hormonal balance of a Stress-Resister returns to normal, urges to eat and to have sex return to pre-stress levels. Stress-Resisters feel like their "old selves again."

The Stress-Resister's hormonal system of checks and balances works well when stressful situations occur only rarely, endure for a short time, and are not extreme in the threat they present.

When faced with unusually intense, repeated, or ongoing stress, however, even the most balanced of Stress-Resisters can be turned into Stress-Responders.

*Although you were born with the body of a Stress-Resister,*
*too much stress can turn you into a Stress-Responder.*

If a stressful experience is extraordinarily strong, if it continues without letup (chronic), or if additional stressors follow within a short time frame, the Stress-Resister's body *learns* to expect stress and remains ready with a new flood of stress hormones poised for release.

This hormonal readiness can color the way that benign, nonstressful situations are perceived, making them appear as if they are far greater challenges. In the face of a perceived threat, once again, the stress-ready body releases stress hormones and the process begins anew. In this way, a cycle of stress perpetuates itself.

# STRESS-RESPONDERS: A BREED APART

Stress-Responders react quickly and with great sensitivity to the world around them. By their nature, Stress-Responders often try too hard, give too often, put their own needs on hold, and care too much. Whether they wish it or not, their bodies are built to more fully and swiftly sense the environment and respond to it.

In prehistoric times, Stress-Responders would have been the greatest of hunters, the most sensitive of caretakers, the problem solvers, heroes, and leaders of the clan.

In today's world, however, Stress-Responders struggle to survive in a sea of imbalance and disconnection. Their senses are assaulted by a myriad of overpowering, unpleasant, or potentially unhealthy experiences. They have little time to consider or evaluate. Their thoughts may become fragmented and reactive. Their bodies can be overtaxed.

Stress-Responders are caught in a world for which their bodies were never intended. Their very genetics makes them less able than others to ignore the torrent of demands that surround them. They are natural stress-eaters.

*Given the right environment, Stress-Responders*
*are almost certain to become stress-eaters.*

Stress-Responders are endowed with trigger-quick hormonal reactions. More than 20 years ago, scientists reported that genetic differences predisposed some individuals to be more responsive than others to stress, especially to mental demands or social stress (Horikoshi et al., *American Journal of the Medical Sciences*, 1985).

In the 2 decades since that discovery, hundreds of scientists have confirmed that an individual's genetic predisposition can make one person a "high responder" to stress and another a "low responder" (Kudielka et al., *Psychoneuroendocrinology*, 2009; Kabbaj, *Archives of Neurology*, 2008).

Stress-Responders have been shown to ignore a negative experience when their stress hormone levels are low but to become fixed on the same negative experience when their stress hormone levels are high; this is a reaction not typically seen in their low-responder counterparts. The difference in responders appears to be strongly connected to genetic differences (Roelofsa et al., *Biological Psychiatry*, 2007).

Early experiences, especially childhood trauma or neglect, can have a strong hand in determining who will become a Stress-Responder as well (Pervanidou, *Journal of Neuroendocrinology*, 2008; Weissbecker et al., *Psychoneuroendocrinology*, 2006).

> *It's not all genetics. Young children who are exposed*
> *to powerful or ongoing stressful situations*
> *are almost certain to become Stress-Responders.*

Whatever the cause, genetic or environmental, Stress-Responders often disregard their own emotions until their needs can no longer be put on hold. Desires, hopes, and dreams are often abandoned under the weight of never-ending demands.

Though they try hard to please others, to take care of family and friends, and to prove their worth, Stress-Responders may experience emotional overload or burnout and find themselves isolated from the world at large, from those who have meant the most to them, and eventually from themselves.

Stress-Responders feel stress more intensely than Stress-Resisters because their bodies are being stressed to a greater degree by hormonal changes. Stress-Responders may wonder how Stress-Resisters can be so unconcerned about so many things. Stress-Resisters, on the other hand, may not be able to fathom why Stress-Responders get so involved, why they care so much, or why they try so hard.

In reality, both Stress-Resisters and Stress-Responders have little choice in the matter. They are simply reflecting differences in their bodies' hormonal responses to stress.

While others may be able to shrug off the abuses and frustrations of modern-day life, Stress-Responders are hardwired to react, to try to bring balance to the outside world in the same way that their bodies require it within. The stress hormones their bodies release are intended to impel them to take action. When no action is taken, the stress hormones are caught in the bloodstream with no place to go.

> *A Stress-Responder's level of stress hormones can be*
> *2 to 10 times greater than those of a Stress-Resister.*

This hormonal excess, well known to scientists, drives Stress-Responders to seek food—carbohydrate-rich and/or high-fat foods, in particular—in a vain attempt to bring their hormone levels, and their bodies, back into balance.

Within moments of eating or even smelling or seeing high-carbohydrate and/or high-fat foods, however, a Stress-Responder's body begins to release high levels of insulin, which in turn signals the release of a surge of cortisol along with other stress hormones.

This repeated and responsive release of hormones is called Stress-Eating Rebound (or Cortisol Rebound). When it is coupled with stress-eating, it can keep a Stress-Responder on a hormonal roller coaster . . . indefinitely.

# 7

# The Stress-Eating Cycle

We've all been taught that stress, overeating, and excess weight can lead to bodies that are unhealthy and lives that are unhappy. In the Stress-Responder, however, a far more powerful chemical change takes place. If you're a Stress-Responder, stress, overeating, and excess weight can lead to Stress-Eating Rebound, a physical response that can pull you into an overwhelming, almost inescapable cycle of stress-eating.

*If you're in Stress-Eating Rebound, your stress hormones increase, rather than decrease, after a snack or meal.*

After eating, Stress-Resisters are likely to feel calm, satisfied, and content. Chances are, they will feel that way for several hours or more.

On the other hand, Stress-Responders, having consumed a meal or snack that they hoped would reduce their stress, may find themselves in the throes of a hormonal hurricane. Surges of cortisol and insulin lead to blood sugar spikes and plunges. Adrenaline surges through their bodies, making their hearts race in a fearlike response. They may find themselves suddenly devoid of all energy and seek sleep in what could only be described as a postmeal stupor.

Even if Stress-Eating Rebound is not severe, it is likely to leave Stress-Responders feeling more anxious, emotional, hungry, and unhappy than they had been before eating.

*The greater the feeling of relief after the first bite of food, the greater the hormonal imbalance.*

While the signs of postmeal Stress-Eating Rebound are obvious, one telltale sign of Stress-Eating Rebound can often be experienced in the very first bite the Stress-Responder takes.

If, in that first bite of carbohydrate-rich and, often, high-fat food, you experience a sense of relief, as if you had been holding your breath waiting for that first bite, it is pretty certain that you are responding to hormonal imbalance and that Stress-Eating Rebound is almost certain to follow. The sense of relief is the result of being rescued, by the consumption of food, from a form of chemical withdrawal. Clearly, it is no surprise that this food is fondly referred to as Comfort Food.

## THE COMFORT FOOD CATCH-22

There is good reason why stress-eaters turn to Comfort Food when they feel tense or anxious. The most common reason given is that it tastes good, of course.

Yet, the same food carries the same taste sensation at nonstressful times; and, though the same food may be eaten at nonstressful times, it is often *not* eaten with the same intense need. Nor is the pleasure that is experienced as great.

*The Comfort Food you reach for may be your body's attempt to get things back in balance.*

If it's not the taste that stress-eaters seek, why do they repeatedly return to Comfort Food?

Only recently have researchers begun to explore the remarkable ability of some people to instinctively attempt to bring balance to their stressed hormonal systems by reaching for Comfort Food.

Drs. Dallman, Pecoraro, and their colleagues, reporting in *Proceedings of the National Academy of Sciences*, describe the power of stress hormones to set up a "chronic stress-response network" in which the pleasure of sweet and high-fat foods "motivates the ingestion of 'Comfort Food.'"

"We propose," they conclude, "that people eat Comfort Food in an attempt to reduce the activity in the chronic stress-response network with its attendant anxiety."

And it appears that Comfort Food works!

"There is no doubt that eating high-fat and carbohydrate Comfort Foods cheers people up and may make them feel and function better," these scientists conclude. "In the short term, or in societies where there is not immediate and continual access to Comfort Foods, occasional relief of anxiety with sweet or fatty foods is probably useful." But, they add, as we all know too well, the habitual use of Comfort Foods "may make one feel better, but it is likely to be bad for long-term health."

So, if you think you've been reaching, without thought, for Comfort Food, consider that something in you has instinctively been trying to make things right with your hormones!

*Stress-Eating Rebound feels as if you're going through withdrawal—because you are.*

Unfortunately, for Stress-Responders, the comfort is usually temporary, and, with the advent of Stress-Eating Rebound, they can find themselves in an ever-deepening withdrawal, needing more comfort than they did at the start, and caught in a seemingly inescapable Stress-Eating Cycle.

## THE STRESS-EATING CYCLE: A CRASH COURSE

The Stress-Eating Cycle is a repeating, almost unbreakable cycle of Stress-Eating Rebound that, if not corrected, will feed into itself indefinitely.

Take one hormonal system that has been genetically programmed or trained to repeatedly overproduce hormones, and add the stimulation of available and highly palatable food.

To this ready mix, add a frustrating, frightening, demanding, or highly unpleasant experience; a generous sprinkling of social pressure; high performance expectations; and a good portion of self-blame. Voilà! The Stress-Eating Cycle is born!

*The hormones that follow cortisol control your cravings, your hunger, and your weight.*

Cortisol, the master stress hormone, is the first to respond to stress, and it will keep the cycle going as well. In order to get its work done, cortisol commands other hormones to do its bidding. This mighty hormone can easily increase levels of insulin and ghrelin, two equally powerful hormones that regulate cravings and hunger and tell your body that it must have food. With similar ease, cortisol can decrease levels of serotonin and leptin, two hormones associated with satisfaction and weight-loss regulation that will no longer indicate when it's time to stop eating and, likewise, will no longer signal your body to burn fat.

When levels of cortisol are low and your body needs food, you feel hungry—naturally—and satisfied when you've eaten enough. When levels of cortisol are high, however, or when they keep peaking, you are almost certain to feel hunger and cravings even when you don't need food; and you may rarely, if ever, get the signal to stop eating.

It is no wonder, then, that the Stress-Responder, caught in a cycle of stress-eating, releasing higher and higher levels of cortisol and its helper hormones, will, almost certainly, fall into a cycle of stress-eating that feels almost impossible to escape.

## PUSHED PAST THE LIMIT

The body has its limits. When the Stress-Eating Cycle continues too long, when the body is able to sense that its own well-being is in jeopardy, the Stress-Responder's overtaxed hormonal system does what it must do to survive: It shuts down.

In this case, shutting down is the body's way of reducing stress, breaking the Stress-Eating Cycle, and resetting itself. The medical term for this shutdown is *adrenal fatigue*.[1]

Stimulating experiences of any kind hold little interest, sleep (though it may be troubled) is greatly desired, and any activity that requires effort is avoided.

---

[1] There may be many causes of adrenal fatigue of which stress-eating may be contributory as only one. Only the appropriate medical professional can advise as to the correct diagnosis and treatment of this condition.

*Adrenal fatigue can be seen as your body's desperate attempt*
*to bring your hormones back in balance.*
*There are far better ways to get the job done.*

For the Stress-Resister, adrenal fatigue is likely to be accompanied by a decrease in cortisol along with a rebalancing of insulin, ghrelin, serotonin, and leptin. When all goes as it should and the Stress-Eating Cycle is broken, the experience of hunger and satisfaction returns to normal.

In the Stress-Responder, however, a different scenario takes place. Though cortisol levels drop, the Stress-Responder, already acclimated to high stress levels, may unknowingly take action to keep the Stress-Eating Cycle in motion.

By continuing to eat foods that stimulate insulin release and, in doing so, keep cortisol, ghrelin, serotonin, and leptin levels out of balance, the Stress-Responder continues to experience intense and recurring cravings without the respite of satisfaction. In a similar way, a tendency toward negative thinking—constantly finding fault with one's self, one's weight, and with others, for example, or feeling inappropriate levels of frustration at even the smallest of annoyances—can be the body's way to keep the cycle going.

*The Stress-Eating Cycle feeds itself . . . literally.*

## DAMNED IF YOU DIET, DAMNED IF YOU DON'T

Though some Stress-Responders, through sheer determination and willpower, may succeed in resisting their hunger and cravings, they still may remain caught in the Stress-Eating Cycle.

Fighting off the body's compelling impulses to eat may be experienced as stress; and this stress, like any other, causes the release of the very hormones that bring with them surges of stress-hunger, cravings, a drive to stress-eat, and weight gain.

Though they succeed in resisting compelling impulses to eat, these determined Stress-Responders may, nevertheless, experience intense cravings and weight gain—even as they are faithfully adhering to their various weight-loss programs.

*Blaming yourself for your eating or your weight*
*could help make you fat.*

In addition, when Stress-Responders make negative judgments about their eating behaviors, weight, appearance, or lack of willpower, it is no wonder that they can remain trapped in a Stress-Eating Cycle for life.

## ADDING INSULT TO INJURY

Cortisol adds one final punch to the very Stress-Eating Cycle that it fuels. Even as Stress-Responders successfully fight off the stress-hunger and cravings that urge them to eat excessively, through a complex set of chemical commands, cortisol signals their bodies to store, as fat, the energy it extracts from whatever meager bits of food they eat.

*Your love handles and tummy fat may come more*
*from the stress in your life than from the food.*

When cortisol levels are high, fat is stored as abdominal fat—the form of weight gain that poses the greatest health risk.

Not all stress-eaters respond in the same way to cortisol's fat-storing power. You may watch helplessly as your weight goes up even though you've been eating no more than usual. Or, trying hard to lose weight, you may experience maddening weight-loss plateaus. You may have been able to lose weight but remain unable to lose the excess fat you hold around the middle. Or, you may have endured it all.

At times, the sheer frustration of fighting one's own body can make any attempt to lose weight seem like a useless battle. And it will remain a no-win situation as long as you *fight* your body instead of *using* its hormonal system to help set you free.

The *way* in which you will use your body to break free of stress-eating is simple! It depends on only one question: What *kind* of stress-eater are *you*?

# 8

# The Stress-Eating Quiz

## *How Strong Is Your Stress-Eating Drive?*

No two stress-eaters are alike. Some may experience only occasional stress-eating episodes, while others may be caught in a Stress-Eating Cycle so frequently that it may feel as if there is no breaking free.

The greater the hormonal imbalance, the more frequent, intense, and enduring your stress-eating episodes are likely to be.

*Your body is unique in every aspect.*
*The way it responds to stress is*
*as individual as your fingerprints.*

## THREE KEYS TO FREEDOM

In order to break the Stress-Eating Cycle permanently, you will need to learn more about three things that are unique to you.

1. How strong is your stress-eating drive?

2. Which hormones are out of balance?

3. What is the best way to bring your particular hormonal imbalance back into balance?

The answers to the first two questions will determine the answer to the third.

The Stress-Eating Quiz that follows on the next page will help you determine the answer to the first of these questions—the strength of your stress-eating drive. The answer to this first question is important because the greater your stress-eating drive, the greater your hormonal imbalance.

In the quiz that follows, you will be asked 18 questions, and depending on your responses, you will discover if you are likely to have a Doubtful, Mild, Moderate, or Strong Hormonal Imbalance.

With an understanding of the strength of your hormonal imbalance in hand, you'll be ready to discover which hormones are out of balance (your Stress-Eating Type) and to get on your Stress-Eating Cure Program.

# THE STRESS-EATING QUIZ INSTRUCTIONS

1. Please take the test when you are alone. It should be completed at one sitting. Until you have scored the test, please do not discuss the questions with anyone else.
2. For each of the questions, answer "YES" if the question is usually true and "NO" if it generally is not true. Answer every question.
3. Answer each of the following questions as if you were *not* holding back on your eating or dieting.
4. Answer each question as if it stands by itself.
5. Trust yourself and your own perceptions. There are no "right" or "wrong" answers.

# THE STRESS-EATING QUIZ

## How Strong Is Your Stress-Eating Drive?

For each of the questions, answer "YES" if the question is usually true. Answer "NO" if it generally is not true.

1. There are times when I eat, or continue to eat, when I'm not hungry.

2. On occasion, either while I'm eating or not long after I finish eating, my heart begins to race.

3. Sometimes I continue to eat food that I am not really enjoying that much.

4. About an hour or two after eating a full meal that includes dessert, I sometimes want a snack or another dessert.

5. At times, I get a sleepy, almost "drugged" feeling after eating.

6. I have a hard time going to sleep without a bedtime snack.

7. At times, I have bitten into my food in anger or have eaten with the thought of "getting back" at someone.

8. Sometimes, while I'm eating, I tell myself that I'm going to stop, but I keep on eating.

9. If I am feeling irritable or edgy, a snack often makes me feel better.

10. In the past, I have done well on a diet until faced with a stressful situation.

11. On occasion, I have eaten to the point of physical discomfort.

12. Once I begin to eat sweets or starches, junk food, or snack foods, I have a difficult time stopping.

13. I sometimes feel as if eating is the only real pleasure I can count on in my life.

14. There have been times when I have continued to eat even though I was upset with my eating or worried about my weight.

15. Often, by midafternoon, I hit a "low" period and feel tired and/or sleepy.

16. I have hidden food, hidden evidence of my eating, or eaten in secret.

17. I have made repeated promises to myself or others that I will take control of my eating and/or my weight, but I have been unable to keep my promises for more than a short time.

18. At least one of my blood relatives suffers from (a) obesity, (b) diabetes, (c) alcoholism, and/or (d) stress-eating.

    *(For this question only, add one point for each of the four different types of disorders in your family. If one family member has*

*more than one disorder, add a point for each new disorder. Maximum points for this question: 4)*

# SCORING THE STRESS-EATING QUIZ

1. Score 1 point for each "YES" answer (0 points for "NO").

2. Question #18 score will be 0–4 (as indicated).

3. Add up all points, then read "What Your Score Indicates" below.

TOTAL: _____ (Total Possible Score: 21)

# WHAT YOUR SCORE INDICATES

## How Strong Is Your Stress-Eating Drive?

Your stress-eating drive is the direct result of the level of your hormonal imbalance. The greater your hormonal imbalance, the stronger your drive to stress-eat and the more often you will experience its power.

**DOUBTFUL IMBALANCE:** Free of Stress-Eating (1–5 points)

**MILD IMBALANCE:** Occasional Stress-Eater (6–10 points)

**MODERATE IMBALANCE:** Recurring Stress-Eater (11–15 points)

**STRONG IMBALANCE:** Frequent Stress-Eater (16–21 points)

# UNDERSTANDING YOUR SCORE

## Doubtful Hormonal Imbalance

### Free of Stress-Eating (1–5 points)

A score of 5 or less suggests that if, at times, you lose control of your eating and/or have difficulty keeping your weight down, your problems do not appear to be related to a hormonal imbalance that we recognize or an ongoing stress-eating problem. If these problems continue, however, it is important to look elsewhere to determine their cause.

# Mild Hormonal Imbalance

### The Occasional Stress-Eater (6–10 points)

Your score indicates that you have a Mild Hormonal Imbalance that, occasionally, drives you into a Stress-Eating Cycle. Some Occasional Stress-Eaters find that they may eat out of habit, when they aren't really hungry or craving anything in particular. At other times, they may eat in response to stress, anxiety, or to meet the increased demands of activity (more to come on this in Chapters 9 through 20).

Occasional Stress-Eaters usually have only mild or moderate weight problems. They may have concerns about gaining weight as they age or become less active.

Many Occasional Stress-Eaters are dissatisfied with their undisciplined eating habits. They may wish they ate less junk food and fast food, and fewer sweets.

Though Occasional Stress-Eaters may not, as yet, exhibit severe weight or health problems, ongoing poor eating habits, forthcoming significant stressors, and the simple act of aging may lead to an increase in stress-eating frequency and intensity.

When faced with situations that worsen their particular kind of hormonal imbalance, including injury, illness, financial or social problems, or other highly stressful challenges, Occasional Stress-Eaters may move to a Moderate or Strong Imbalance and discover an increase in weight- and health-related problems.

*If you have a Mild Imbalance, you may think*
*that all you need to do is try a little harder. Wrong!*

The real problem with having a Mild Hormonal Imbalance is that it's easy to convince yourself that, if you just tried harder, you could get your eating under control.

Actually, the opposite is true. When stress-eaters with a Mild Imbalance force themselves to try to follow traditional low-calorie or other restrictive eating programs, they can set themselves up for even greater stress-eating challenges.

Dieting deprivation can push a mildly out-of-balance hormonal system over the edge and kick it up to a Moderate Imbalance. The negative feelings that come with failing at dieting or with gaining even more weight can kick it up a notch once again.

Countless well-meaning, Occasional Stress-Eaters with only Mild Hormonal Imbalances have ended up in far worse straits because they simply didn't know that their problem was physical and, clearly, not a matter of willpower.

## Moderate Hormonal Imbalance

### The Recurring Stress-Eater (11–15 points)

Your score indicates that you have a Moderate Hormonal Imbalance that repeatedly propels you into a Stress-Eating Cycle.

Recurring Stress-Eaters move in and out of their respective Stress-Eating Cycles. At times, they may convince themselves that uncontrolled eating is normal. At other times, they become greatly concerned over their lack of control, weight, and health.

Recurring Stress-Eaters may experience persistent hunger or cravings for Comfort Foods (carbohydrate-rich and/or high-fat foods). Impulses to eat these foods may shift from mild to overpowering. The intensity of the hunger and cravings can make consistent, good eating habits and weight control almost impossible. Sometimes, Recurring Stress-Eaters may show signs of future weight problems, though clearly this is not always the case.

Recurring Stress-Eaters may not understand why there are times when they are well able to control their impulses to eat or snack while, at other times, this control simply slips away. Often, they do not realize that their ability or inability to control their eating springs from the highs and lows of a fluctuating hormonal imbalance.

*Moderate Imbalance?*
*For you, control comes and goes.*

Spouses, family, and friends of the Recurring Stress-Eater may try to be sympathetic. Their support, however, may not be sincere and enduring. At times, friends and family have witnessed the Recurring Stress-Eater in full control of his or her eating. They may assume, therefore, that control is always an option. Due to the lack of understanding that, for some, stress-eating is a recurring (and not consistent) disorder, Recurring Stress-Eaters are often wrongly judged and misunderstood.

When faced with future ongoing or highly stressful situations specifically keyed to their particular patterns of hormonal imbalance (as you will see in Chapters 9 through 20), Recurring Stress-Eaters may be at increased risk for weight- and health-related problems.

# Strong Hormonal Imbalance

### The Frequent Stress-Eater (16–21 points)

Your score indicates that you have a Strong Hormonal Imbalance that drives you into a Stress-Eating Cycle and may, at times, prevent you from escaping.

The majority of stress-eaters are unhappy with their eating and/or their weight. Often, they are at a loss as to how they can help themselves. In addition to frequent weight concerns, they may experience an inability to concentrate, mood swings, anxiety, and/or lack of motivation.

From past experience, Frequent Stress-Eaters have discovered that even their best efforts to control their eating are undermined by recurring and intense stress-hunger and cravings.

*Strong Hormonal Imbalance? Deprivation diets will spike your cravings*
*and bring your metabolism to a grinding halt.*

Any period of "healthy eating" or dieting for weight reduction is doomed to be short-lived and followed by failure. Frequent Stress-Eaters live with feelings of frustration and concern. When they are kept too long from the foods they crave, the hormonal imbalance that drives their stress-hunger urges them to give in and give up. To make it even harder, high levels of cortisol can prompt higher levels of insulin, bringing their ability to lose weight to a standstill.

The excess of stress hormones that surge through their bodies can interfere with the Frequent Stress-Eaters' abilities to think clearly, creating an experience that some describe as a *brain fog* (especially after eating). Frequent Stress-Eaters may feel isolated or abandoned. Worse, they are almost certain to blame themselves.

In the future, as stressful experiences particularly relevant to the Frequent Stress-Eater's pattern of stress-eating present themselves (as detailed in Chapters 9 through 20) or as age-related changes worsen their hormonal imbalance, Frequent Stress-Eaters are at increased risk for weight- and health-related problems.

## WHO IS THE STRESS-EATING CURE PROGRAM FOR?

The Stress-Eating Cure Program has been designed for Occasional, Recurring, and Frequent Stress-Eaters with Mild, Moderate, and Strong Hormonal Imbalances, respectively. If you are a stress-eater, it will offer you the means to eliminate your stress-hunger, cravings, stress-eating, and weight problems without struggle.

## A QUESTION OF WEIGHT

There is no absolute correlation between your weight and your level of stress-eating. Although the more frequently you are caught in a Stress-Eating Cycle, the greater the *likelihood* that you will gain weight, this is not always the case.

If your score indicates that you are a Recurring or Frequent Stress-Eater and your weight falls within a normal weight range, one can assume that your natural metabolic rate or your level of activity is causing your body to burn excess energies at a very fast rate. If that same level of stress-eating continues, however, and you are faced with a decreased level of activity; with unexpected, prolonged, or intense stressors; or with the simple act of aging, you may be faced with more severe weight problems.

*Being slim doesn't protect you*
*from stress-hormone-induced health problems.*

Even though slim Recurring or Frequent Stress-Eaters do not carry the burden of extra pounds *as yet*, they can suffer the same increased health risk that overweight stress-eaters experience. Correcting the underlying hormonal imbalance is important to their health and longevity even if weight may not be a primary concern.

## IMPORTANT NOTES

Before beginning the eating portion of the Stress-Eating Cure Program, read Chapters 9 through 20. In these pages, you'll discover which hormones are most likely to be responsible for your particular pattern of stress-eating, which triggers are most likely to set off a Stress-Eating Time Bomb, and what you can do to stop your Stress-Eating Cycle before it even gets started.

# PART
# III

# 9

# What Type(s) of Stress-Eater Are You?

What do the following things have in common?

> Skipping breakfast
>
> Repeated dieting
>
> Diet drinks
>
> Regular mealtimes
>
> Lack of sleep
>
> Natural flavorings in your food
>
> Overweight friends
>
> A difficult childhood
>
> Certain types of viruses
>
> Sitting at a computer or desk for most of the day
>
> Aggravating friends or family
>
> The lack of gentle and loving touching
>
> Many antidepressants, antihistamines, birth control pills, and high blood pressure and migraine medications

The answer? Depending on *your* particular Stress-Eating Pattern, any of the Stress-Eating Triggers above can lead to an onslaught of stress-hunger, cravings, stress-eating, and weight gain.

Your score in the Stress-Eating Quiz (Chapter 8) revealed the *strength* of your drive to stress-eat. In that chapter, you learned that the strength of *your* drive to stress-eat differs greatly from that of other people.

In this chapter, you will discover that the *types* of stressful situations that trigger your stress-eating can differ greatly from those of other people as well.

When faced with impossible demands or intense pressure, for example, you may experience intense stress-hunger and cravings, while a friend may experience a drive to stress-eat only when faced with an uncomfortable social situation. Indeed, no two stress-eaters are exactly alike.

> *When it comes to stress-eating, one-size-fits-all doesn't work.*
> *To stop stress-eating and lose weight, you need a program*
> *that addresses your individual differences.*

## STRESS-EATING PATTERNS: WHEN TRIGGERS SEIZE CONTROL

What makes one person react strongly to an impossible work demand and another barely react to it? Why does an argument with a family member send you running for a snack, yet have a very different effect on the person with whom you are arguing?

Researchers have discovered that slight imbalances in your hormone levels can greatly affect the type of situations that trigger you to stress-eat.

Your body's hormonal balance or imbalance is the result of three influences: your genetics, your past experiences, and the day-to-day situations in which you find yourself. This unique mix of nature and environment directs your body to respond to certain things in the world around you and to ignore others. Those situations or experiences that lead to stress-hunger, cravings, stress-eating, and weight gain, we term Stress-Eating Triggers.

If, for example, you were raised in a home in which it was essential to please your parents and, in addition, your genetics determined that you were, by nature, sensitive to the facial expressions, tone of voice, and comments of others, you would find it difficult to ignore little things that others barely notice. In response to the stress of being on guard and constantly evaluating your behavior and that of others, your body could be expected to experience an onslaught of stress hormones when faced with a social situation; this surge of hormones would be many times that which another person might produce in a similar setting. The cascade of hormones you experienced could be expected to repeat, more quickly and with greater intensity, each time you encountered a social situation.

Depending on a stress-eater's particular genetics and history, other types of hormonal overreaction can result from a wide variety of other Stress-Eating Triggers: family responsibilities, work demands, time and money constraints, loss of affection or companionship, unexpressed anger, anxiety, lack of sleep, and more.

Stress-Eating Triggers, as well as the hormones they summon, vary from individual to individual, but one rule remains unswervingly in place: Your hormones have been designed to take control of your actions and to stay in control.

*Your body is being shaped, literally,*
*by the hormones surging inside you.*

When released, each hormone rewards you with a strong sense of pleasure when you follow the impulses it stimulates. Likewise, each produces an even stronger sense of discomfort when you do not comply. While feelings of anxiety, irritability, restlessness, the inability to concentrate, a sense of impending doom or panic, or a generalized negativity may be caused by a variety of factors, often they are the price our hormones extract when we resist their demands to eat in response to stress.

If that weren't challenging enough, consider the following: When two or more stress hormones are in play at the same time, they can form a powerful partnership that translates into almost undeniable impulses. Willpower is virtually useless against these biochemical urges. The only way to break a hormone's powerful grip is to disarm it at its foundation. Once you know which hormones you're fighting, the solution falls easily into place.

Most Stress-Eating Triggers fall naturally into one of 11 types, called Stress-Eating Patterns. Each Stress-Eating Pattern can include many triggers that are similar in their cause and in the hormones that they are likely to stimulate. All of the triggers within each particular Stress-Eating Pattern are experienced in a similar way and are likely to be associated with the same basic underlying hormonal imbalance that is likely to lead to stress-hunger, cravings, stress-eating, and weight gain.

## THE SCIENCE BEHIND THE CURE

For decades scientists have been documenting and exploring the hormonal changes that determine which Stress-Eating Patterns are likely to pull you into their control.

*Emotions and hormones are a two-way street.*
*Each can cause great changes in the other.*

At one time, an individual's feelings and perceptions were considered to be the *cause* of hormonal changes. Anxious about something? It's no wonder your adrenaline is peaking, you'd be told. Most recent research, however, has revealed that the reverse is just as likely to be the case. Scientists now understand that, in many cases, our feelings and perceptions are quite likely to be greatly influenced as a *result* of the hormones that surge within.

Here is just a small sampling of what scientific research has revealed about the hormones that underlie the top Stress-Eating Patterns.

Tension, depression, anger, confusion, and fatigue were significantly greater among subjects in whom cortisol levels were brought to highest points (re: Anxiety-Induced Stress-Eating or Avoidance-Induced Stress-Eating Patterns).

—F. Martin del Campo et al., *Biological Psychiatry,* 2002

Hostility, cynicism, and aggression were found to increase as levels of adrenaline were increased (re: Self-Sacrificing Stress-Eating, Frustration-Induced Stress-Eating, and Secret Stress-Eating).

—Richard S. Surwit et al., *Psychosomatic Medicine,* 2009

Low oxytocin levels resulted in greater anxiety and lowered levels of interpersonal attachment (re: Avoidance-Induced Stress-Eating).

—Mattie Tops et al., *Psychophysiology*, 2008

Raising levels of insulin significantly increased feelings of anger, despite the fact that subjects were in a non-confrontational setting (re: Carbohydrate-Induced Stress-Eating and Guilt-Induced Stress-Eating).

—McCrimmon et al., *Physiology and Behavior*, 1999

In the past, virtually all weight-reduction programs have failed because they did not recognize the following essential facts about stress-eating.

1. Stress-eaters are driven to eat by triggers in their environment that set off hormonal imbalances.

2. Triggers generally fall into one of 11 Stress-Eating Patterns, each containing its own unique set of hormonal imbalances.

3. When a stress-eater's Stress-Eating Pattern is identified and treated accordingly, stress-hunger, cravings, stress-eating, and weight problems literally disappear.

# THE DISCOVERY

These three essential facts were unknown to us when we began our research. Our goal was simple: to develop a treatment for stress-eating that would correct the cause of stress-related hunger, cravings, and weight gain. It was important to us, as well, that the treatment would result in a struggle-free and deprivation-free cure for those who found themselves caught in stress-eating's powerful grip.

At first, we assumed that stress-eating was a single entity with a single cause and a single cure. We searched amid the thousands of pages of our research subjects' detailed daily logs for clues to the cause of a stress-eater's hunger, cravings, and compelling need to eat.

One fact quickly became clear to both of us, however; no *single* cause could account for the wide variety of triggers that set off stress-eating episodes among our subjects.

With that understanding firmly in place, we reexamined the data from a completely different vantage point. We sought patterns of internal and external triggers, environmental stresses, feelings, thoughts, and experiences that predictably led to stress-eating—different combinations for different subjects.

The multitude of daily logs that our subjects completed provided our first clues. Research subjects had been required to keep real-time records of the intensity and frequency of their hunger and cravings; the date, time, quantity, quality, and source of their food and drink; and their moods, physical and/or emotional experiences and thoughts, throughout the day and evening, in response to external stresses, prior to eating, and in response to eating. In addition, they kept records of their activities, medications, and changes in medical status, and detailed records of their daily weights and weekly averages.

From this rich source of data, we found statistically significant relationships and patterns, cause-and-effect connections that predicted stress-eating episodes.

Isolating the triggers that would predict stress-eating was an important first step. Determining the causes, explaining *why* different patterns of stress-eating occurred, however, was an entirely different matter. It was made especially difficult because the causes were, most likely, nearly impossible to measure and document.

This is the scientific challenge that researchers have encountered for centuries. Five hundred years ago, Nicolaus Copernicus hypothesized that, contrary to popular belief, the sun did not revolve around the earth but, rather, the other way around. With no way to measure the movement of the earth and sun and prove his hypothesis, Copernicus did the next best thing: He predicted that *if* his hypothesis were correct, certain events could be expected. His ability to correctly forecast the position of celestial bodies verified his hypothesis although no physical proof was available.

In the same way, long before Pasteur's Germ Theory was accepted, he proved that invisible microorganisms were the cause of fermentation, spoilage, and disease by designing experiments that prevented the result by removing the cause.

Galileo, Einstein, and countless others have employed similar methods with similarly accurate results.

Today's forensic scientists use the same method to postulate the actions of a criminal who no one has observed but whose existence is almost certain in light of the impact on the crime scene.

So it goes with each of the hormonal imbalances that we postulated were the cause of the variety of Stress-Eating Patterns we observed.

In the dynamic living body, it is virtually impossible to measure hormones with any consistency or accuracy. Hormonal levels change from moment to moment; measurements of hormones in urine differ in magnitude and consistency from those in the saliva. No standardized tests can be counted on to document average levels according to gender, age, weight, and genetic predisposition.

How then could we document the array of hormonal imbalances that were causing the Stress-Eating Patterns we had observed?

The answer: First, by describing and predicting the observable stress-eating patterns that one would expect if, indeed, a distinct set of hormonal balances did exist and, second, by eliminating stress-eating in each of those patterns by applying treatments specifically designed to alter their respective hormonal imbalances.

Using the behaviors and emotional experiences unique to each Stress-Eating Pattern that we had observed in our research subjects' logs, we sought all relevant hormonal connections reported in the scientific literature.

Fortunately, many of the behaviors and emotions that we were researching had been linked, repeatedly, to a discrete set of hormonal imbalances. We identified those hormonal imbalances that were most likely responsible for the behaviors and emotions that were being reported among our subjects. In addition, in many cases, we were able to confirm that the most effective treatment strategies reported by our research subjects (and readers, as well) were connected to these same hormonal imbalances.

The next 9 years were spent confirming and refining the cause and effect of ever-changing hormonal imbalances that, by their nature, defied standardized measurement.

Treatment strategies were tested, adapted, and tested again for their ability to stop stress-eating and bring about struggle-free weight loss for each of the 11 Stress-Eating Patterns.

Detailed daily logs and weight charts documented the effectiveness of each treatment strategy for each Stress-Eating Pattern. Only those that offered consistently significant amelioration of stress-hunger, cravings, stress-eating, and weight problems were included in the Stress-Eating Cure Program.

Each of the Stress-Eating Patterns that you are about to discover reflects a different hormonal imbalance as researched above. The strength, ease, and effectiveness of the Stress-Eating Cure Program lies in the fact that it was designed just for you, for your Stress-Eating Pattern. By eliminating the specific hormonal imbalance that is driving your stress-hunger, cravings, and weight gain, the Stress-Eating Cure Program, along with the individualized recommendations to come, will help you break free of your Stress-Eating Pattern.

The Stress-Eating Patterns in the chapters to come include:

The Frustration-Induced Stress-Eater

The Social Stress-Eater

The Self-Sacrificing Stress-Eater

The Secret Stress-Eater

The Carbohydrate-Induced Stress-Eater

The Anxiety-Induced Stress-Eater

The Task-Avoiding Stress-Eater

The Guilt-Induced Stress-Eater

The Exhaustion-Induced Stress-Eater

The Quicky Stress-Eater

The Delayed Stress-Eater

After only a quick glance, you may be pretty certain that you already know which Stress-Eating Pattern(s) describe(s) you best. Still, we urge you to read through all of the Stress-Eating Pattern chapters that follow. Some are almost certain to surprise you!

In combination, these Stress-Eating Pattern chapters will:

1. Help you determine your Primary Stress-Eating Pattern

2. Help you discover which hormones are driving your particular Stress-Eating Pattern

3. Provide you with individualized recommendations for turning the basic program into your personalized Stress-Eating Cure

If, as you read, you notice that more than one Stress-Eating Pattern seems to describe you, you're probably right on target. Stress-eaters move through different patterns throughout their lifetimes and can alternate between two or more patterns at the same time.

Read through each chapter description, and, in the end, one Stress-Eating Pattern will almost certainly emerge as your primary Stress-Eating Pattern: that which *best* describes you! Armed with an understanding of *your* body's hormonal imbalance, you'll be ready to get started on the program and find the freedom from stress-eating that you have sought for so long.

# ALL THAT YOU NEED

## Rachael:

When I was 38 years old and still weighed more than 300 pounds, I had a recurring dream. In the dream, I stood outside a shop, looking with longing at a woven, orange straw rug. In the dream, I desperately wanted to own it, but I knew it was beyond my means. Still, I would stand outside the window, looking at it and imagining that it was mine.

One night, the last night that I had the dream, I decided to go into the shop to see if I could work out a way to purchase it. The woman in the shop said little but indicated that I should look closer at the rug. When I did, I discovered that there were many areas that appeared black among the woven straw.

I indicated that I was surprised and dismayed at the black areas I had never noticed before. The shop owner smiled and revealed a secret.

"Those are not black areas among the color," she explained. "They are areas that are not yet complete. But," she added, with a knowing nod, "you have everything you need to complete it."

It was then that I knew that the slim, healthy, normal body and the freedom from cravings that I longed for were well within my reach. I needed only to be willing to learn all that I still needed to know and apply that which I had learned.

## Rachael and Richard:

In the pages that follow, you will discover all that you need to stop stress-eating and get control of your eating, your weight, and your life. You hold the cure in your hands. It works if you work it, and it's here, waiting for you, in the chapters that follow.

*You hold in your hands all that you need.*

This program comes with a wish from both of us—the heartfelt hope that you will let go of the defeats of the past; that you will embrace the idea that although you have been wronged, blamed for a physical disorder, a victim to an undiagnosed and untreated hormonal imbalance, there is an answer that can bring you the freedom you have been waiting for.

Come fresh to this program; allow yourself to know that, all along, it was *not* your fault! Allow yourself to know that you were right to keep searching for an answer and that, finally, you have found it.

# 10

# The Frustration-Induced Stress-Eater

Imagine, for a moment, that you are trying your best to get a job done: an assignment at work, a task at home, or a personal project. It might be quite complicated or something as simple as changing a doctor's appointment. But you keep hitting the same problem: the incompetence, irresponsibility, or plain old stupidity of the people you have to deal with. Or you might be thwarted by an absurd impenetrable automated phone system that won't allow you access to a human being who would get you what you need.

More and more often, your mate, family, friends, co-workers, and the world at large astound you with their ignorance, ineptitude, and blatant lack of concern. Your own abilities and hard work are consistently blocked by a world that is going downhill . . . fast. Getting anything done, much less done right, is getting far more difficult, if not impossible. At times, you are simply fed up with the world and sick of fighting.

This is the daily experience of the Frustration-Induced Stress-Eater. On a regular basis, Frustration-Induced Stress-Eaters are forced to deal with people and situations that they perceive as irritating or aggravating. The world fails to live up to their expectations and often thwarts their best efforts.

Most Frustration-Induced Stress-Eaters have a field of reference that is different from the situation in which they currently find themselves. Chances are, they were raised in an environment that demanded competence and responsibility. Or they remember a world in which courtesy and a reasonable work ethic were the rule rather than the exception. In either case, they find themselves "strangers in a strange land" of inadequacy, absurdity, and impossibility.

Frustration-Induced Stress-Eaters often feel that people and circumstances beyond their control keep them from meeting demands and expectations (their own as well as those of others).

*Frustration-Induced Stress-Eaters may feel as if everyone and/or everything is getting in their way.*

It is at these times—when they are held back from getting something done or done right—that Frustration-Induced Stress-Eaters often feel as if they are fighting the world. They may vacillate between feelings of exasperation and powerlessness. If you are a Frustration-Induced Stress-Eater, you probably take great delight when you are finally able to take control of a situation and make it "right." When you find yourself helpless to change things for the better, however, your emotions may trigger stress-hunger and cravings that are hard to escape, even after the problem person or situation is no longer an issue.

*Frustration-Induced Stress-Eaters are caught in a two-way hormonal battle for control.*

When you are hit by cravings or stress-hunger, you are probably experiencing the combined impact of high levels of adrenaline and low levels of oxytocin.

Oxytocin, the hormone of affection, bonding, and sexual arousal, is released in response to your body's nurturing and sexual feelings. When oxytocin is high, you experience a sense of closeness, comfort, and love. When it is low, these feelings can quickly disappear.

Oxytocin, and the loving feelings that it brings, plummet in the face of stress. Cortisol, released in response to a stressful situation, causes your adrenaline levels to rise. The higher the levels of adrenaline, the lower the levels of oxytocin. The more stress, the less the feelings of love and connection.

Oxytocin, however, is pretty powerful in its own right. It has the ability to decrease adrenaline as well. As with many other hormone pairs, these two are in a never-ending battle for control of your feelings.

Imagine oxytocin in one corner, growing stronger in response to a loving touch or word, or from natural, sexual changes within your body. Now, picture adrenaline in the other corner, trying to push away your loving feelings and replace them with feelings of aggression and power.

These two fighters remain in an ongoing battle for control of your feelings. The food you eat, the beverages you drink, and almost every action you take determine which will have the advantage.

*You've probably been using one hormone*
*to control the other for a long time!*

When you've sought comfort in the arms of someone you love, when a conversation with a good friend has made you feel less worried, when just watching your children sleep has wiped away some of the tensions of the day, you have used oxytocin's power to reduce adrenaline and the unpleasant feelings of stress that accompany it.

You've experienced the opposite action in those moments when worries about family matters or a disagreement with your mate has wiped away your desire to make love, when lingering work pressures caused you to snap at your child or mate, when a noisy, hot, or unpleasant environment made you testy with those closest to you. At those moments, you've experienced adrenaline's power to decrease your levels of oxytocin.

Under ideal circumstances, this give-and-take of hormones works well, but when stress is ongoing or recurring, oxytocin's levels may drop too often and remain low too long. If stresses remain high, you may not realize that the hormonal battle within you may be causing you to feel lonely, easily irritated with those you love, or disconnected from feelings of affection.

Low levels of oxytocin can impact your stress-hunger and cravings and cause you to want to eat . . . and eat . . . and eat. The medical term for this unbridled intake of food is *hyperphagia,* and in many cases it is related to low levels of oxytocin.

Although many stress-eaters experience the challenges that come from occasional high levels of adrenaline, Frustration-Induced Stress-Eaters carry the added burden of these levels remaining out of balance for long periods of time.

To make matters even more difficult, adrenaline has been shown to decrease the body's sensitivity to insulin so that the food that is eaten in response to oxytocin-induced stress-hunger and cravings is almost certain to end up as fat, most likely to be deposited around the middle.

You've probably seen sitcoms that portray the heroine digging into a quart of ice cream after being dumped by her boyfriend or in anticipation of some nerve-racking event. These scenes simply dramatize low levels of oxytocin in action.

In an unconscious attempt to raise their oxytocin levels, Frustration-Induced Stress-Eaters often gravitate toward smooth and creamy foods such as chocolate, pizza, and Chinese food. Sharing a meal with someone else, however, can raise oxytocin levels and naturally reduce the desire for food. Since being in the company of others can raise oxytocin levels, Frustration-Induced Stress-Eaters often eat less when eating in a social environment.

Frustration-Induced Stress-Eaters rarely take the time to cook meals for themselves, unless they are cooking for others at the same time. In other ways, as well, Frustration-Induced Stress-Eaters often put others' needs before their own. When they encounter a world in which their needs or preferences are given minimal consideration, the feelings of frustration can feel overwhelming. In such a hormonal cycle, stress-eating is all but inevitable.

## YOUR PERSONALIZED PLAN

To help eliminate stress-hunger, cravings, stress-eating, and to lose weight and keep it off, Frustration-Induced Stress-Eaters need a Personalized Plan designed to decrease the levels of adrenaline that flood their bodies. At the same time they need help in boosting their levels of oxytocin. This combination of hormone-balancing goals is a great deal easier to attain than you might think.

# GETTING STARTED

In Chapter 30, The Frustration-Induced Stress-Eater's Cure, you will find simple, effective recommendations that are individualized specifically for the Frustration-Induced Stress-Eater. Read through Chapter 30 and apply the tips you find there to the Stress-Eating Cure Program (Chapters 21 through 29). These personalized suggestions will help turn the Stress-Eating Cure Program into your personalized Stress-Eating Cure.

# 11

# The Social
# Stress-Eater

Picture yourself surrounded by food, friends, and fun. Sounds like a good time, right? Now, consider that while you are in the midst of conversation, a part of you notices that you are consuming foods that you don't want to be eating. You know that your weight—even your health—may suffer, but you feel helpless to stop.

You try to comfort yourself with thoughts that the social situation is time-limited and that as soon as you're alone once again and able to focus, you'll get your eating back under control. Or you might justify your unchecked eating spree as a well-deserved splurge and, again, promise yourself that when alone you will go back to "being good."

Chances are, however, that when you are alone, you will find that you're still unable to get a grip on your eating. And so the Social Stress-Eating Cycle begins.

*The food doesn't have to be great or the company terrific
to set off a Social Stress-Eating Cycle.*

The food that triggers the Social Stress-Eater does not have to be hugely desirable nor the people in the social situation of particular importance. The combination of the proximity of food along with the potential of positive reinforcement that derives from intimate experiences is enough to cause hormonal levels to rise and fall rapidly.

Social situations and the availability of food lead Social Stress-Eaters to surrender to the pleasures of the moment, while concerns about diet and weight fleet or fade. Though they may not know it,

Social Stress-Eaters are not exhibiting a lack of willpower but, rather, simply following the path that their hormones have laid before them.

It's likely that you've experienced Social Stress-Eating when you've been so involved in a conversation that you barely tasted the food you were putting in your mouth. Or, at other times, you might have eaten hors d'oeuvres or other finger foods at a social occasion and realized too late that you had been so busy in conversation that you had eaten far more than you had intended.

Social Stress-Eaters often feel as if a distant part of them is urging them not to eat too much but that they lose focus on that intention. Instead, they get "lost" in a conversation or are distracted by the chaos of a party or dinner.

Some Social Stress-Eaters find that restaurants are their downfall. Often, they find themselves caught between wanting to control their eating and the temptation of ordering the foods they really want. Phrases such as "Just this time," "It's only one dinner," "I deserve it," or "After all, it's a celebration" give Social Stress-Eaters a reason to indulge the powerful impulses that urge them to eat. Other Social Stress-Eaters are embarrassed to order a "diet meal" and prefer to avoid the risk of being cross-examined as to their weight-loss progress.

*You may offer up many reasons for Social Stress-Eating,*
*but, chances are, it's all a matter of hormones.*

No matter what the rationale Social Stress-Eaters may come up with, most likely it is their underlying hormonal imbalance that is driving their desire to eat.

The combination of socially stimulated stress-hunger, cravings, and stress-eating, which is the hallmark of the Social Stress-Eating pattern, comes from the interplay of two hormones.

Oxytocin, the hormone of affection, sexual arousal, and bonding, rises quickly in positive social situations. High levels are reached in response to the body's sexual and nurturing feelings.

When oxytocin levels soar, adrenaline levels plummet—as does self-restraint. As long as adrenaline remains low, Social Stress-Eaters find little need or desire to focus on anything but the social situation on hand. With weight-loss goals no longer a top priority, they continue to eat, drink, and make merry.

## WHEN IS A SOCIAL STRESS-EATER NOT A SOCIAL STRESS-EATER?

The answer is simple! If you are *not* enjoying the company, if you are wishing you could avoid or escape the social situation, or if you are desperately desirous to get away and, instead, find yourself diving into food . . . you are *not* engaged in Social Stress-Eating.

*Did you enjoy the social contact?*
*What you feel makes all the difference.*

Your stress-hunger, cravings, and stress-eating may arise in the middle of a social situation, but if you are *not enjoying* the social connection, the Social Stress-Eating experience has been turned into a Frustration-Induced Stress-Eating experience (see Chapter 10). Rather than wanting to relax and linger over the interpersonal connection (as a Social Stress-Eater would), you want out!

## YOUR PERSONALIZED PLAN

Social Stress-Eaters tend to surround themselves with an ongoing flow of friends. By taking refuge in social situations, they give themselves license to eat without restraint. In Chapter 31, The Social Stress-Eater's Cure, you will find simple, effective recommendations that are individualized specifically for the Social Stress-Eater. Read through Chapter 31 and apply the recommendations you find there to the Stress-Eating Cure Program (Chapters 21 through 29). These personalized suggestions will help turn the Stress-Eating Cure Program into your personalized Stress-Eating Cure.

# 12

# The Self-Sacrificing Stress-Eater

In an early Hindu myth, Purusha, a primal being, sacrifices himself so that creation can take place. His eye becomes the sun, his head the sky, his breath the wind, and so on. Purusha is honored for his acts of sacrifice that keep the cosmos stable. In a similar vein, the mythology of the Aztecs includes a central tale of two gods who formed the universe by splitting a goddess in half so that one part of her became the sky and the other part became the earth. For centuries, her followers honored her sacrifice.

Likewise, modern-day Self-Sacrificing Stress-Eaters may feel as if they're being torn apart by the demands of the world around them and that their sacrifices are necessary to keep all in working order. Their offerings, however, are far less likely to be honored or even acknowledged.

While one may never know if the figures of mythology gave of themselves with enthusiasm, clearly this is not the case for Self-Sacrificing Stress-Eaters who experience stress rather than satisfaction as they meet each new demand.

Self-Sacrificing Stress-Eaters are givers—not by nature, but rather by necessity. They are the fixers, those who can be counted on to save the day, to take up the slack left by those far less capable or responsible.

Their actions are motivated by necessity, not altruism. Experience has taught them that if they don't do the job or take on a responsibility, no one will. Alternately, they have come to understand that if someone else does it, it won't be done well. Or, even worse, that in the end, other people's incompetence will mean more work for them.

Not surprisingly, Self-Sacrificing Stress-Eaters are often competent. When they do a job, they do it well. Often they may discover, however, that their successes lead not to a respite from demands and pressure but instead to ever-more-demanding responsibilities.

*The world of the Self-Sacrificing Stress-Eater*
*can be a lonely one. The more they give,*
*the less they seem to get.*

The payoff for their hard work and commitment is often far less than that which Self-Sacrificing Stress-Eaters might hope. In most cases, their hard work and willingness to help are taken for granted. Their competence and care are rarely given the recognition or the appreciation they so clearly deserve.

As a result, Self-Sacrificing Stress-Eaters often feel the need for just a bit of compensation. In general, the few moments of pleasure Self-Sacrificing Stress-Eaters desire is little enough reward in exchange for the time and energy they offer up in the service of others.

*Though they more than deserve the little pleasure*
*they seek, their reward comes at a price.*

The problem, however, lies in the fact that Self-Sacrificing Stress-Eaters are often so starved for a few moments of pleasure or reward that any bit of relief they experience is likely to send them into a whirlwind of desire. With the first comfort-filled bite of carbohydrate-rich or high-fat food, the Self-Sacrificing Stress-Eater is often pulled into a Stress-Eating Cycle that can feel like both a blessing and a curse. A blessing because of the extraordinary pleasure that Comfort Foods bring; a curse because, once enjoyed, the reward of Comfort Foods can make other pleasures or the satisfaction of a job well done seem unimportant.

The hormonal imbalance that triggers this onslaught of stress-hunger and cravings for the Self-Sacrificing Stress-Eater is triggered by a combination of high levels of adrenaline and low levels of the pleasure hormone, dopamine.

Adrenaline is released, or overreleased, when high levels of cortisol, the master stress hormone, are released. Adrenaline is the hormone of action. It is the body's way to motivate you to get what you need for survival. Unfortunately, adrenaline is also released when you only *think* or *feel* as if your well-being were in jeopardy.

Loud noises can be perceived by the body as a threat; overcrowded situations, emotional confrontations, the anticipation of a confrontation, any of a thousand everyday occurrences can trigger a cortisol release followed by an adrenaline rush.

There are some adrenaline rushes that can feel pleasurable; a great deal depends on the state of mind and the way in which your particular genetics set you up to interpret the experience. A free fall on a roller-coaster, for example, is a thrilling experience for one person and a dreaded horror for another. Whatever the feeling, adrenaline has one main purpose: to get the body all that it needs to handle the stress or threat that it faces (or believes it is facing).

When a fresh rush of adrenaline surges through your bloodstream, it signals your liver to make more blood sugar available to your brain and muscles. While some people appear to want less to eat when their adrenaline levels begin to rise, it appears that the opposite is true when adrenaline levels remain high for a prolonged time.

If you are a Self-Sacrificing Stress-Eater, you are likely to experience an uneasiness, an undirected arousal, when adrenaline levels remain high. You may feel that you need to do something, though you're not certain what that something is.

As long as adrenaline levels remain high, you will continue to seek something to bring your body back into balance. Top priority on that list of necessities is usually food, primarily in the form of blood sugar.

*Adrenaline rising short-term can mean no desire to eat.*
*Adrenaline remaining high can mean the desire*
*to stop eating disappears.*

You may have experienced the difference between the first rush of adrenaline and chronically high levels yourself. It's often experienced when an unexpected or stressful situation wipes away all thought of food only to be followed, after a while, by an intense desire to eat.

Some researchers have wondered why adrenaline would prompt you to eat when you are in the midst of a fight-or-flight situation. Others have hypothesized a logical answer: When the stressful situation continues, it is important to replenish the food supply. When stress does not quickly disappear, your body calls other hormone helpers into action, including insulin and additional cortisol, great hunger-makers in their own right.

The Self-Sacrificing Stress-Eater can be pulled to overeat even though there is no real threat or stress to the body. When there is no immediate problem to deal with, high levels of adrenaline can stimulate the mind to look for a problem to solve. Like a carpenter with a hammer in hand, you may find yourself on the lookout for any nails that might need a good slam.

Unfortunately, when you are in that state of arousal, each new problem you focus on and solve, or focus on and are unable to solve, raises your adrenaline levels higher. And so, particularly for those who are genetically sensitive to adrenaline's effects, a self-perpetuating cycle is created.

For the Self-Sacrificing Stress-Eater, this cycle can present a challenge because high levels of adrenaline combine with low levels of dopamine.

*Adrenaline and dopamine: hormones on a seesaw.*

Dopamine transmits messages in the brain and, in many ways, is similar to adrenaline. Among its other jobs, dopamine affects cells that control emotional responses and the ability to experience pleasure. When your dopamine levels are low, you may feel *blah*; when you feel intense pleasure, it is likely that your dopamine levels are spiking.

The types of triggers that cause our bodies to release dopamine are as varied as our preferences and genetics. Whatever brings intense pleasure your way is your path to dopamine release.

Dopamine is a building block for adrenaline; when adrenaline is first being made, excess dopamine is called into action and may be more readily available to bring sensations of pleasure. Over time, however, high levels of adrenaline interfere in two ways with dopamine's ability to make you feel good.

First, when most of your body's dopamine is used in the making of adrenaline, less remains for other functions, such as experiencing pleasure. Second, adrenaline competes with dopamine at the doorways, or receptor sites, to nerve cells that can transmit pleasure.

Adrenaline acts like the school bully, hogging all the food in the lunchroom for himself and blocking the doorway when other kids want to go to their classrooms. As long as adrenaline continues to block dopamine from making the right connections in the brain, the Self-Sacrificing Stress-Eater experiences recurrent feelings of longing for any of a thousand sources of emotional or physical pleasure or spiritual joy. Self-Sacrificing Stress-Eaters seek comfort in food, but that comfort is fleeting because their dopamine stores are low and their ability to experience pleasure is hampered. The cycle is vicious and hard to beat.

*Balance the adrenaline levels that are keeping you*
*from experiencing pleasure, then sit back*
*and let your body feel good—all over.*

# YOUR PERSONALIZED PLAN

You might be tempted to assume that indulging in more pleasurable activities will bring you the rewards you seek. Ironically, indulging in pleasurable activities is *not* likely to bring any additional pleasure to the Self-Sacrificing Stress-Eater. The excitement associated with most pleasurable activities is likely to raise adrenaline levels even higher. As long as adrenaline levels remain high, dopamine is likely to be used to fuel the cycle of adrenaline-making, leaving little left over for the experience of pleasure or satisfaction.

If there have been times when you have wondered why few things seem to bring you pleasure anymore, don't worry! We've got the answer *and* the solution.

*Your lowered ability to feel real pleasure*
*or experience deep satisfaction may be little more*
*than a matter of hormones!*[1]

---

[1] The diminished ability to experience pleasure or satisfaction can be indicative of more serious biochemical imbalances that require professional intervention. In all cases, be guided by your physician's recommendations.

The good news is that if you're a Self-Sacrificing Stress-Eater, there's an easy way to bring pleasure back into your life and experience the feelings of joy and satisfaction you so richly deserve.

The Personalized Plan for Self-Sacrificing Stress-Eaters in Chapter 32, along with the Stress-Eating Cure Program itself (Chapters 21 through 29), will guide you each step of the way.

In Chapter 32, The Self-Sacrificing Stress-Eater's Cure, you will find simple, effective recommendations that are individualized specifically for the Self-Sacrificing Stress-Eater. Read through Chapter 32 and apply the recommendations you find there to the Stress-Eating Cure Program. These personalized suggestions will help turn the Stress-Eating Cure Program into your personalized Stress-Eating Cure.

# 13

# The Secret
# Stress-Eater

Standing in the glow of an open refrigerator, you gulp down the food you've been waiting to get to all evening, alert to any sound that might indicate someone from the next room is about to enter. Just in case, you have a plan in place: Should anyone interrupt your stolen moment of pleasure, you will simply take a swig from the open bottle of water you have ready and swallow all evidence of your crime.

Secret Stress-Eaters may feel that they are fooling those closest to them, hiding the depth of their stress-hunger, cravings, stress-eating, and weight problems (as much as possible), but this very isolation creates greater stress, which, in turn, feeds into the hormonal imbalance that rules their eating and their lives. They live in a world of isolation and shame.

More than almost any other Stress-Eating Pattern, there is a very clear set of feelings and behaviors that define the Secret Stress-Eater. Although you don't have to experience *all* of the signs of Secret Stress-Eating to confirm a diagnosis, a Secret Stress-Eating Pattern is likely if you have experienced three or more of the following:

1) a preference to eat alone (even though the same foods may be enjoyed in the company of another)

2) the consumption of large quantities of food in a short period of time

3) an excitement in anticipation of a secret-eating event

4) hoarding and/or hiding of food

5) feelings of irritability or frustration if an eating event is interrupted or must be postponed

6) anxiety, fear, or a physical or emotional reaction to the thought of being discovered

If you are a Secret Stress-Eater, you may experience the last of these signs—an anxiety or fear of being discovered—as the opposite emotion. Although many Secret Stress-Eaters may be upset at the mere thought of being discovered by a mate, family member, or friend, at times there may also be an unrecognized desire to *get revenge* or *get even* with another, a desire for Secret Stress-Eaters to prove that they will not be controlled.

*Hormones run wild in the bloodstream*
*of the Secret Stress-Eater.*

This ambivalence between wanting to tell the world that you are an independent individual with a right to some pleasure in combination with feelings of guilt, shame, and fear of repercussions, is enough to send adrenaline levels through the ceiling. Add to this mix insulin spikes that come from carbohydrate-rich foods—that is, the foods most easily eaten in secret—and you get the high-adrenaline, high-insulin combination that defines the Secret Stress-Eater.

This same imbalance can keep the Secret Stress-Eater in its grip indefinitely. To make matters worse, if you are a Secret Stress-Eater you are almost certain to gain weight as time goes on. As the patience of friends, family, and mates is pushed to the limit by unfulfilled promises, you may find yourself becoming even more resentful.

Now, with the stakes even higher, adrenaline levels can reach all-time peaks. You are more likely to eat intensely sweet or rich foods in secret and with more frequency. Insulin levels climb to even greater heights. Though you've done nothing but respond to your body's over-powering messages, it is only a matter of time before you may find your health—your physical and/or mental well-being—hanging by a thread.

*Almost any stress-eater can become trapped*
*in a Secret Stress-Eating Pattern.*

## YOUR PERSONALIZED PLAN

So, what can be done to break Secret Stress-Eating's powerful hold? The answer surprised us. You'll find it in full in Chapter 33, The Secret Stress-Eater's Cure.

## GETTING STARTED

In Chapter 33 you will find simple, effective recommendations that are individualized specifically for the Secret Stress-Eater. Read through Chapter 33 and apply the recommendations you find there to the Stress-Eating Cure Program (Chapters 21 through 29). These personalized suggestions will help turn the Stress-Eating Cure Program into your personalized Stress-Eating Cure.

# 14

# The Carbohydrate-Induced Stress-Eater

Starches, junk food, snacks, and sweets. Imagine that, to you, they are not simply pleasurable indulgence, but rather a powerful matter of need. When you take your first bite of carbohydrate-rich food after not having had any for a few hours, your body experiences profound relief, as though you'd been holding your breath until that moment.

That first bite, like the first drink for an alcoholic, sets off a drive to eat that is virtually unstoppable. With your first forkful of pasta, your first bite of pizza or a chocolate éclair, the creamy first taste of ice cream or cheesecake, you are hooked. No matter how many times you promise yourself that you'll eat just a little or in moderation, when the food hits your mouth, it's as if an "on" switch has been thrown and you simply cannot stop.

Rather than feeling satisfied, you find that the more you eat, the more you want. If, for instance, you have breakfast, you generally find that you are hungrier before it's time for lunch than if you had had nothing but a cup of coffee.

People who are *not* Carbohydrate-Induced Stress-Eaters cannot even imagine how someone could be hungrier a few hours after eating breakfast than if they did not.

The reason you experience this post-carbohydrate hunger can be summarized in one word: *insulin*.

*It isn't necessarily the food you're eating for breakfast
that's affecting you but, rather, what you ate last night.*

When Carbohydrate-Induced Stress-Eaters consume a full breakfast after eating carbohydrate-rich foods the night before, insulin levels spike, blood sugar levels go haywire, and stress-hunger and cravings can become overpowering.

Eating carbohydrate-rich foods late in the evening readies the body to release extraordinarily high levels of insulin if carbohydrate-rich foods are eaten again in the morning.

Among scientists, this phenomenon is called the Second Meal Effect. This effect demonstrates the power of the food you eat at one meal to influence your body's reaction to the same food many hours later. Both the cause and correction of the Second Meal Effect are defined by the excess levels of insulin that shape a Carbohydrate-Induced Stress-Eater's most intimate experiences and greatest challenges.

Carbohydrate-Induced Stress-Eaters are the quickest of all types of stress-eaters to put the blame on themselves. At times, their stress-hunger and cravings may be five times stronger than those who have no underlying hormonal imbalance. Still, most Carbohydrate-Induced Stress-Eaters assume everyone experiences the same intense carbohydrate-hunger and cravings as they do.

Nothing could be further from the truth! In a wide variety of laboratory mice and rats, several different forms of genetic combinations determine that some animals will become obese and some will not, even though they are fed and exercised in exactly the same way. These fat-destined animals overproduce the fat-making hormone, insulin, in response to frequent meals of carbohydrate-rich or high-fat foods.

Left to their own devices, these adorable, fat-destined rodents will eat excessively, gain weight, and exhibit much of the same hormonal imbalances as their human counterparts. Even when they are not given free rein to extra food, their bodies will still make fat from what little food they do consume.

No one would ever think to blame these little round rodents for a lack of willpower. Clearly, the animals' genetics are the cause of their excess hunger and their increased ability to turn food into fat.

*Obesity, diabetes, and alcoholism have more in common*
*than you might suspect. And it's all in the genes.*

It should come as no surprise, then, that Carbohydrate-Induced Stress-Eaters often have a family history of obesity (sometimes along female lines only), adult-onset diabetes, and/or alcoholism: three closely connected diseases of metabolism. In our article entitled "The Genetics of Obesity" in the *McGraw-Hill Encyclopedia of Science and Technology,* we reviewed the discovery of several genetic forms of obesity and the hormonal imbalances that are the hallmark of these disorders.

Most common of all of these genetic disorders is the imbalance that has come to be known as Carbohydrate-Induced Stress-Eating or Carbohydrate Addiction.

*Addiction: When you aren't doing it, you wish you were.*
*When you are doing it, you wish you weren't.*

The reason that we've used the term *addiction* is simple: In keeping with the World Health Organization's definition—which involves (a) repeated use of a substance, (b) difficulty in voluntarily ceasing or modifying its abuse, and (c) the willingness to obtain the substance by almost any means—the appropriateness of the word *addiction* seems obvious. At least it does to most carbohydrate addicts.

In less scholarly terms, we define *addiction* as an action that when you're *not* doing it, you wish you *were*. And when you *are* doing it, you wish you *weren't*.

The reason for including this disorder as a Stress-Eating Pattern comes from the understanding that, for those who have this genetic predisposition, carbohydrate-rich foods are experienced by the body as a stress-filled challenge—especially when these foods are eaten frequently or in unbalanced meals.

*You are not to blame for your carbohydrate addiction,*
*but there are many things you can do to break free.*

The good news is that when it comes to Carbohydrate-Induced Stress-Eating, your genetics are not destiny. As you will discover in this chapter, in the Stress-Eating Cure Program, and throughout this book, the *way* in which you take in your carbohydrate-rich foods can make all the difference in the world.

When Carbohydrate-Induced Stress-Eaters feel the urge to stress-eat, they are responding to their bodies' high levels of insulin. Insulin is your body's fat-making hormone. Among its many jobs, it is responsible for taking food energy from your bloodstream and bringing it into the muscles, nerves, and organs that need it for fuel.

When all goes right, insulin helps move just the right amount of blood sugar from the food you eat to where it is needed most, throughout your body. If a little food energy—in the form of blood sugar—is left over, insulin helps move it into the liver, where it is turned into blood fat and stored away in the fat cells. Insulin works this magic by acting like a gatekeeper, opening tiny doorways (called *receptor sites*) that allow the energy to move into cells.

After a few hours, when blood sugar levels drop, insulin levels fall as well. Other doorways open and allow the fat to leave the fat cells so that the muscles, nerves, and organs can burn up the bit of excess fat that has been stored away.

When too much insulin is produced, however, the system goes a bit haywire. At first, excess insulin permits too much blood sugar to flood the muscles, nerves, and organs, and Carbohydrate-Induced Stress-Eaters may feel energized by a carbohydrate-rich meal of starches, snack food, junk food, or sweets. The excess food energy that they may have taken in is ushered to the liver to be turned into blood fat and stored away. Carbohydrate-Induced Stress-Eaters may notice that they gain weight easily. But since consuming carbohydrates leaves them feeling so good, they may still be quite active or involved in an exercise regimen (which helps burn excess energy and bring insulin levels back into balance). They may be able to keep their weight somewhat under control.

*Your body defends itself against too much of*
*a good thing in the only way it can.*

Over time, however, it becomes increasingly difficult to keep insulin's power under control. In addition to its fat-storing ability, insulin has the ability to strongly stimulate the desire to eat carbohydrate-rich foods and to make those foods taste exceptionally delicious.

Without an eating program that helps correct the insulin imbalance, carbohydrate-rich foods are eaten more and more frequently and in less balanced meals, and higher insulin levels flood the body. Muscles, nerves, and organs begin to sense a need to defend themselves from this flood of insulin and blood sugar, and the doorways to these tissues begin to shut down. They actually disappear!

With few places to take its load of blood sugar, insulin signals the liver to turn more of the excess energy into fat and to store great quantities in the fat cells, more fat than the body will ever be able to burn.

*Carbohydrate-Induced Stress-Eaters are starving*
*even as they are gaining weight by leaps and bounds.*

Carbohydrate-Induced Stress-Eaters experience this second stage of hormonal imbalance in two ways. First, they often notice a pronounced tiredness, lack of energy, or desire to be active. With so little energy feeding their muscles and nerves, it is no wonder that they are tired.

Second, they are almost certain to see their weight skyrocket. They may blame their weight gain on their lack of activity, but, in reality, both the lack of energy and the weight gain are coming from a tsunami of food energy that insulin has directed to be siphoned into the fat cells.

In the third and final stage of Carbohydrate-Induced Stress-Eating, even the fat cells begin to sense a need to defend themselves against insulin's overpowering energy-hoarding ability. The doorways to the fat cells close down and disappear as well.

With little energy going to the fat cells, the Carbohydrate-Induced Stress-Eater stops gaining weight or may begin to lose weight. This is not a *healthful* weight loss but, rather, the result of the body's inability to take fat into the fat cells. With no place to go, the fat remains in the bloodstream, a most dangerous condition.

Now, insulin's power has reached a dead end. The Carbohydrate-Induced Stress-Eater is said to be "insulin resistant." With no place to go, blood sugar levels continue to rise, signaling the official start of the disease we call adult-onset diabetes.[1]

*You can harness insulin's power to help eliminate
stress-hunger, cravings, and weight concerns—for life.*

There is no doubt that without an understanding of insulin's power and an awareness of how to break its stranglehold, Carbohydrate-Induced Stress-Eaters are almost certain to watch their eating and weight spin out of control and their health deteriorate. There is, however, no doubt that the reverse is true as well!

## YOUR PERSONALIZED PLAN

When a few simple guidelines are put into place, insulin's power is easily harnessed and used for good. You will be able to enjoy the carbohydrate-rich foods you love every day while getting and keeping control over your eating and your weight.

## GETTING STARTED

In Chapter 34, The Carbohydrate-Induced Stress-Eater's Cure, you will find simple, effective recommendations that are individualized specifically for the Carbohydrate-Induced Stress-Eater. Read through Chapter 34 and apply the recommendations you find there to the Stress-Eating Cure Program (Chapters 21 through 29). These personalized suggestions will help turn the Stress-Eating Cure Program into your personalized Stress-Eating Cure.

---

[1] Adult-onset diabetics must consult the appropriate healthcare professional for approval and supervision prior to making any dietary and/or exercise changes in their regular routine.

# 15

# The Anxiety-Induced Stress-Eater

Consider what it's like to have a mind that is rarely at rest and that often feels as if something terrible could happen at any moment. Anxiety-Induced Stress-Eaters seem to carry the weight of the world on their shoulders. Many live in a world of extremes: too many demands, too little time, too little praise offered too rarely.

Often, they live with an almost never-ending internal tension, a disquiet that can be far greater than any single issue at hand. Recurring dreams may include being in a runaway car or showing up for a school exam without preparation.

*Anxiety-Induced Stress-Eaters may feel as if*
*they are drowning in one crisis after another.*

Some Anxiety-Induced Stress-Eaters may focus on one concern, then, shortly after that issue is resolved, find that another problem emerges. Some Anxiety-Induced Stress-Eaters may juggle multiple demands, each of which is in itself more than any one person can handle. Even when they are not actually fulfilling their responsibilities, Anxiety-Induced Stress-Eaters feel they must make certain all goes as it should.

When Anxiety-Induced Stress-Eaters feel the urge to stress-eat, they are responding to their bodies' high levels of cortisol and adrenaline. Both of these fight-or-flight hormones signal the body to hold onto the energy it may need in preparation for a confrontation or an escape, should either be necessary.

Cortisol is the body's Master Stress Hormone. Imagine it as a general on horseback, readying his troops to go into battle. In preparation for the fight, the general assembles his officers and gives them orders to conserve energy as may be needed in the upcoming fight.

"I'll need a lot of you, Insulin," General Cortisol commands, and the body releases a flood of this hormone. High levels of insulin, in turn, make carbohydrate-rich foods taste particularly good and urge you to ingest as much food as possible.

To ensure that enough food energy is on hand should it be needed, cortisol calls in the hormone ghrelin, which commands you to continue to eat. But cortisol's influence is not limited to these two hormones alone.

Cortisol can decrease hormone levels as well as increase them. When faced with a stressful situation, this Master Stress Hormone decreases leptin levels. Less leptin means a greater appetite and fewer calories burned.

At the same time, cortisol decreases serotonin, the hormone that tells your brain that you are satisfied. This final, double whammy of lower levels of leptin and serotonin makes you want to eat more, leaves you feeling far less satisfied after the meal, and—even as you are experiencing postmeal cravings—makes it almost certain that you'll be turning the food you just ate into fat.

*At least four different hormones urge the*
*Anxiety-Induced Stress-Eater to devour food,*
*then store the food energy as fat.*

As an Anxiety-Induced Stress-Eater, your hormonal imbalance doesn't stop there! High levels of adrenaline urge your body to remain in a fat-making mode and, at the same time, decrease your desire for bonding, sex, and touch by decreasing levels of the hormone oxytocin. Ironically, it is oxytocin and the stress relief this hormone encourages through human contact that are most needed and, sometimes, least desirable to the Anxiety-Induced Stress-Eater.

With all of these hormones urging you to increase your storehouse of energy, it's no wonder that Anxiety-Induced Stress-Eaters often bolt down their food, barely tasting it, rarely chewing it. Anxiety-Induced Stress-Eaters are not overly fussy about food. Although they may have definite preferences, at times Anxiety-Induced Stress-Eaters will eat almost everything that is available. Given the hormones surging within, they have good reason!

# YOUR PERSONALIZED PLAN

## Getting Started

As an Anxiety-Induced Stress-Eater, it is likely you prefer to do something fully and quickly so that you can see immediate results. In Chapter 35, The Anxiety-Induced Stress-Eater's Cure, you will find simple, effective recommendations that are individualized specifically for the Anxiety-Induced Stress-Eater. Read through Chapter 35 and apply the recommendations you find there to the Stress-Eating Cure Program (Chapters 21 through 29). These personalized suggestions will help turn the Stress-Eating Cure Program into your personalized Stress-Eating Cure.

# 16

# The Task-Avoiding Stress-Eater

Picture, if you will, the following scenario: It is 12 o'clock at night and you are seated in front of the computer, barely able to keep your eyes open. Tomorrow morning is the deadline you've been avoiding for 2 weeks. You glance at the clock and a renewed sense of panic grips your chest. For some reason, you simply cannot bring yourself to complete the task that is expected of you.

The job at hand may be a relatively simple task, or it may be so complicated that you don't know where to start. Whatever the level of difficulty, you've been unwilling or unable to face it for days, and it has been hounding you in the back of your mind. Now, there is no way that you can put it off any longer.

Suddenly, you are struck by an undeniable need to eat. You tell yourself that you'll feel better after you've had a snack, that it will calm you down.

When you have finished raiding the refrigerator, you're overcome by a great sense of tiredness. You conclude that, in this condition, you simply cannot concentrate. You lay your head down for only a moment—and the next thing you know it's morning. Clearly, there is no time left to complete the task.

Almost all of us do it from time to time. When it becomes a pattern, your hormones may be calling the shots.

Task-Avoiding Stress-Eating comes in a seeming endless array of types and timings. It may take place when there is no time limit or one that is not close at hand. It may be the result of a job that feels overwhelming, is unpleasant, or is one that you have no reason to avoid.

No matter the cause, Task-Avoiding Stress-Eating serves one major purpose: to keep you from doing what you simply don't want to do.

Some Task-Avoiding Stress-Eating episodes may last only a few minutes and result in a mere stall for time. Other, more extensive food frenzies can result in great physical discomfort or tiredness that temporarily incapacitates the stress-eater, rendering him or her incapable of completing the task at hand.

Task-Avoiding Stress-Eating is more common than you might think. It has been experienced by so many stress-eaters that it might be characterized as a side pattern to most of the other patterns. For those who experience Task-Avoiding Stress-Eating on a regular and frequent basis, however, this pattern of stress-eating can be especially difficult and deserves a place—and a treatment—of its own.

*Task-Avoiding Stress-Eaters can feel helpless,*
*hopeless, and a whole lot more.*

The feelings that accompany Task-Avoiding Stress-Eating have been described in vivid and emotionally revealing ways as "a black hole of fear," "a sort of a paralyzing never-never land," and "a kind of limbo where you know that your life is passing you by, but there's nothing you can do about it." Others have said that, once caught in its grip, the climb out grows steeper by the day until you are certain that there's no way to get back to a productive and peaceful life.

What causes these terror-filled experiences and, more important, what can be done to break Task-Avoiding Stress-Eating's mighty grip?

Task-Avoiding Stress-Eating is the result of high levels of cortisol and low levels of oxytocin. While this hormonal twosome may not seem particularly powerful per se, it is the joint impact of the other hormones this combination calls into action that really packs the emotional and physical wallop!

In the early stages of Task-Avoiding Stress-Eating, high levels of cortisol (the Master Stress Hormone) can rise four to five times that of the average person under stress. This response alone is enough to send your mind and body reeling!

*It's no wonder that you feel overwhelmed!*

In response to moderate stress, your blood pressure can rise. Though you may not be aware of it, your heart may beat more strongly and, most likely, more rapidly as well. You may feel light-headed or experience a sense of nonreality.[1]

As your body is trying to recover its equilibrium, hundreds of other bodily processes are being disrupted by cortisol and the other hormones it has summoned. At cortisol's command, high levels of insulin flood your bloodstream, throwing your blood sugar levels off balance. As your nervous system struggles to get the energy it needs to do its work, you may again experience a light-headedness or an inability to think clearly. Your muscles, unable to get the food energy they need, will likewise begin to conserve energy.

Within moments, you are likely to feel anxious but at the same time depleted of all desire to take action and be unable to focus or think clearly. Like an animal trapped in a cage, you may want to do something, anything, but feel that you are incapable of knowing how to proceed. Everything may seem just too much for you to handle.

As cortisol continues to run unopposed, higher levels of insulin will impel you to eat carbohydrate-rich foods, which, in turn, throw your blood sugar levels even more out of kilter and urge you to continue to eat. High levels of ghrelin are likely to join the chaos, further increasing your hunger by signaling your body that it must have food.

*The anxiety you feel may be an awareness*
*that your hormones are out of control.*

To make matters worse, in later stages of Task-Avoiding Stress-Eating, cortisol can decrease levels of serotonin and leptin, two hormones of satisfaction and weight-loss regulation that will no longer tell you when it's time to stop eating and will stop telling your body to burn fat.

---

[1] All of these conditions may be related to a variety of causes. To determine the correct cause and treatment, it is essential to see an appropriate health care provider.

At the same time, your low levels of oxytocin bring home a second punch. Not only do decreased levels of this bonding hormone make it less likely that you will get the help and comfort you need to break this cycle, they also encourage an increase of the hormone adrenaline. Adrenaline often serves as cortisol's second-in-command, signaling the body and mind that a fight-or-flight response is needed.

In this case, however, your muscles, nerves, organs, and much of the rest of your body have been depleted of the supplies needed to function effectively. Although the message to remain at attention is received, there is little your body or mind can do to offer assistance.

That feeling of helplessness is experienced as an added demand, which creates even more stress and—as you probably guessed it by now—causes the release of more cortisol!

*Most Task-Avoiding Stress-Eaters blame themselves.*
*Wrong, wrong, wrong!*

Most remarkable of all is the fact that with all of the physical and emotional turmoil going on, Task-Avoiding Stress-Eaters are likely to blame themselves for not completing a job or tackling a responsibility.

"Just do it" has become the call of the impossibly demanding world (and some ad campaigns as well). "If I could just do it, don't you think I would?" would be an appropriate response.

Although we would never expect someone with any other handicap to overcome his/her disability at our command, when it comes to hormonal imbalances that play havoc with the mind, body, and will, we expect the impossible.

Task-Avoiding Stress-Eaters face a special challenge not necessarily encountered by other stress-eaters. It is essential that they understand that the difficulties they may have in facing tasks and completing them may be due to the hormonal hurricane that is rampaging through their bodies.

There is good news: When Task-Avoiding Stress-Eaters are given clear, step-by-step guidelines to balance their hormonal imbalances, they can follow them without anxiety; feel relief from cortisol's emotionally overwhelming impact; rediscover their own dreams, desires, and pathways to happiness; and, best of all, take the steps to make their dreams a reality.

So, the next time you feel frozen, unable to confront the overwhelming task(s) that face you, as you strain to find your focus and try to force yourself into action, consider this: With the Stress-Eating Cure, there is an easy passage to the other side of the mountain of anxiety that looms before you.

## YOUR PERSONALIZED PLAN

You have one task before you, and this one will make all of the others to come a great deal easier. Get to know the program that's about to help bring you peace of mind and a slimmer body. Not only does freedom from stress-eating await you but also freedom from self-blame, shame, and fear.

## GETTING STARTED

In Chapter 36, The Task-Avoiding Stress-Eater's Cure, you will find simple, effective recommendations that are individualized specifically for the Task-Avoiding Stress-Eater. Read through Chapter 36 and apply the recommendations you find there to the Stress-Eating Cure Program (Chapters 21 through 29). These personalized suggestions will help turn the Stress-Eating Cure Program into your personalized Stress-Eating Cure.

# 17

# The Guilt-Induced
# Stress-Eater

It's the day after Thanksgiving. Everyone is gathered around the kitchen table, enjoying the leftovers. Suddenly, your least favorite uncle declares he's just remembered that there's a leftover piece of chocolate cake in the refrigerator and heads off to claim it as his own.

He returns a moment later, empty-handed. "Someone ate the last piece of chocolate cake," he declares. Though there are six other people in the room, before thinking, you exclaim, "It wasn't me!"

When something is missing, broken, or has gone wrong, Guilt-Induced Stress-Eaters either feel responsible or are convinced that others assume they are.

Guilt-Induced Stress-Eaters often find themselves in no-win situations. Whatever they do—or don't do—never seems to be quite enough. Not good enough, not special enough, not equal to what they think they could do if they only tried harder!

*The past, present, and future: Each can harbor*
*a different feeling of failure.*

Guilt-Induced Stress-Eaters live in a world of judgment and condemnation that leaves them feeling unworthy and ashamed. Not only do the past and present hold feelings of regret, but fear of future censure or blame leaves them anxious and distressed as well. Whether the feelings of inadequacy focus on gift-giving responsibilities, promises waiting to be fulfilled, obligations, or any of a million daily demands of life, Guilt-Induced Stress-Eaters feel that their inadequacies are obvious and reflect on their intelligence, sophistication, appearance, ability, and/or worth.

Interestingly, when Guilt-Induced Stress-Eaters are asked to examine the thinking behind their feelings of guilt or failure, they often realize the issue of their concern was not as bad as they first thought. The reason for this temporary breakthrough is obvious: It is *not* the situation that intrinsically makes a Guilt-Induced Stress-Eater feel guilty.

In fact, the hormonal imbalance and the amorphous feelings of guilt it produces come first. Once the mind and body are caught in the hold of the combination of high insulin and high oxytocin levels, any problem or concern—related to the past, present, or future—can offer ready-made situations about which to feel bad.

Here's how it works: When insulin levels are high, blood sugar levels are out of balance. The nervous system is either getting too much fuel or too little fuel. In a real, measurable way, it is being irritated. At that point, any action or interaction can become the believed source of the irritation.

In the presence of high levels of oxytocin—the bonding hormone—interpersonal and social experiences take priority. Any small insecurity or concern is likely to become greatly exaggerated.

If adrenaline levels were higher, oxytocin levels might be forced to recede. With little adrenaline to hold back the reins on emotions and blood sugar in full swing, however, feelings of guilt, shame, and regret—real or imagined—go unchallenged. The Guilt-Induced Stress-Eaters' logical thinking can be strongly influenced by their emotions. Though they may *know* they're not to blame, Guilt-Induced Stress-Eaters *feel* guilty just the same.

One of the most important things we have learned in helping people is that feelings aren't facts. It doesn't matter what is or is not true by our standards: If someone *feels* that something is true, at that moment, for him or her, it is true. Furthermore, we *don't* know that they aren't more accurate in their assessment of the situation than are we. So, in truth, we have no right to ever say, "Oh, don't be silly. You shouldn't feel guilty about that!"

*One guilt-filled thought after another.*
*Your hormones are running the show.*

Guilt-Induced Stress-Eaters tend to move quickly from one target of remorse to another. Some may stay fixed on one focus of self-blame. In general, however, Guilt-Induced Stress-Eaters will find that, after a while, one target of concern gives way to another. This is a good indication that a hormonal imbalance is running the show.

Guilt-Induced Stress-Eaters may feel upset all morning at the thought of something they said the evening before. By the afternoon, they may find fault with themselves for the work they failed to finish that morning. With the evening comes an opportunity for self-reproach at having wasted the day.

Also, as evening approaches, a Guilt-Induced Stress-Eater's stress-hunger and cravings often hit—and hit hard. Their bodies have become sensitive to the nightly rise of hormones that are experienced as intense and recurring cravings.

For some, the cravings begin shortly after dinner. An hour or two after the meal is finished, they experience undeniable cravings for something sweet, salty, or crunchy. They may attempt to control their portions but find they cannot resist going back for more.

Feelings of failure at being unable to control their eating add fuel to the fire of self-reproach. Many Guilt-Induced Stress-Eaters pass the rest of the evening vacillating between thoughts of self-condemnation and servings of Comfort Food.

Bedtime can present a special opportunity for guilt gathering. There, in the moments before sleep, the Guilt-Induced Stress-Eater's hormones can reign supreme. In non-stress-eaters, this is a time when insulin levels are low. For the Guilt-Induced Stress-Eater, however, carbohydrate-rich foods eaten throughout the day may result in insulin levels that are three to five times normal. As activity levels subside, already low levels of adrenaline decline. In response, oxytocin levels rise.

*Night-Eating Syndrome is not caused by lack of self-control.*
*It's hormonal, all the way.*

This extreme imbalance can lead to a pattern of Night-Eating Syndrome, a well-recognized condition in which hormonal abnormalities compel the eater to consume great quantities of carbohydrate-rich and/or high-fat foods. Many stress-eaters with Night-Eating Syndrome believe that sleep is impossible if they have not had Comfort Food to quiet their nerves.

There are, however, light, help, and hope at the end of the Guilt-Induced Stress-Eater's tunnel. Although behavioral training, restrictive diets, and psychotherapy may have little impact on the stress-hunger, cravings, stress-eating, and weight gain that plague the Guilt-Induced Stress-Eater, correcting the hormonal imbalance that lies at its heart can make all the difference in the world.

If you are a Guilt-Induced Stress-Eater, learning how to bring insulin and oxytocin levels under control can bring your freedom—for good—on a multitude of levels.

# THE GOLD STANDARD TEST OF GUILT

Guilt is like the air. It's everywhere, so common that it is no longer noticeable. Guilt has become so much the norm that those stress-eaters who are the most dogged by it may be the least aware of it.

As we explained above, Guilt-Induced Stress-Eaters often move from one target of self-blame to another. Not *all* Guilt-Induced Stress-Eaters, however, move from target to target. Some may focus on a single situation or experience and, though their hormones are shaping their feelings, they cannot let go. In this way, their perceptions and emotions may mimic those of someone who is suffering from a real and perhaps justified sense of guilt.

*Is it real guilt or are your hormones talking?*
*It's important to know the difference.*

To help free a Guilt-Induced Stress-Eater from stress-hunger, cravings, stress-eating, and weight gain, it is essential to determine the difference between inappropriate guilt feelings that are *hormone*-driven versus actions or inactions that are more legitimately responsible for evoking guilt.

We need to know the difference to determine if the Stress-Eating Cure Program alone is appropriate. Here's why: When a hormone imbalance alone is the guilt-evoking culprit, the program, in combination with personalized tips and strategies that follow, can quickly and easily bring the Guilt-Induced Stress-Eater freedom from stress-hunger, cravings, stress-eating, and weight concerns.

On the other hand, there are times when an action or inaction may present a legitimate cause for feelings of guilt. If a legitimate guilt-associated action (or inaction) is the cause of the guilt feelings (and the hormone imbalance that can result), additional intervention is required.

We use the following test to help determine if a hormonally based Guilt-Induced Stress-Eating pattern is in play. This exercise, however, is *not* absolute in its accuracy. If you think that a true cause for guilt lies at the base of your Guilt-Induced Stress-Eating or if feelings of guilt persevere, it is essential to obtain professional counseling and support to rectify the situation.

With that said and, we trust, duly noted, here's what we have come to call the Gold Standard Test of Guilt. In a quiet and comfortable situation, we ask the stress-eater to talk to us about his/her feelings of guilt.

If several guilt-related experiences, actions, or inactions are verbalized, we know from the start we are probably looking at hormone-induced guilt feelings (assuming, of course, that the stress-eater is *not* responsible for a myriad of guilt-evoking incidents).

If only one or two incidents are recounted, we continue. When the stress-eater fully communicates the reason for his/her guilt, we restate what we have heard in our own words. Then we ask the stress-eater to describe an alternate scenario that might have resulted from a particular situation, a scenario that could have brought with it a positive outcome.

If a stress-eater feels guilty about nagging her daughter to the point that the young woman quits high school and moves away from home, an alternate scenario might be that the mother's tenacity helped her daughter see the light, straighten up her act, and achieve her potential. We ask the stress-eater to linger a moment, experiencing the feelings associated with the positive outcome.

*You could have done the opposite,*
*and things would have turned out worse.*

Taking a different vantage point, we then ask the stress-eater to imagine that he/she took the opposite action to that which is now evoking guilt. In the case of the nagging mother, we ask her to imagine that she held her tongue. Most stress-eaters can see that an alternate action might have just as well resulted in the same outcome or one that was worse. In the case of the mother, not speaking up could have resulted in the girl's risk-related behavior that could have put the young woman's life in danger.

Finally, we add the perspective of the long view. "What might still happen?" we ask. We remind the stress-eater that in most cases the cards are still in play. The mother might yet get a call from her daughter and learn that, out in the world on her own, the girl realized the value of all that she had left behind; that, with her mother's help, she is ready to return to school and put some energy into making a life for herself.

With all these different scenarios before them, most Guilt-Induced Stress-Eaters realize that their guilt is related to only one of many paths that their actions (or inactions) might have precipitated. If any of these other scenarios might have taken (or might still take) place, they cannot reasonably blame themselves for an outcome.

With this understanding, the true turning point of the Gold Standard Test of Guilt takes place. If the stress-eater carries this understanding to a deeper level and experiences a release from guilt, chances are he/she is a Guilt-Induced Stress-Eater at a low or moderate stage of hormonal imbalance. We suggest that they choose either the Quick-Start Plan or the Step-by-Step Plan of the Stress-Eating Cure Program. Professional counseling may or may not be appropriate.

On the other hand, if the stress-eater immediately jumps to other guilt-evoking targets, it is likely that a full-fledged hormonal tsunami is driving their thinking and their emotions. For these Guilt-Induced Stress-Eaters, the Quick-Start Plan is strongly recommended, as well as professional counseling.

When the Gold Standard Test of Guilt evokes no change in feelings or understanding, there is the possibility that some action or inaction requires professional attention prior to beginning the program. We suggest that stress-eaters seek appropriate counseling. Once the guilt-evoking issue is resolved, the program can be applied to hormone-related hunger, cravings, stress-eating, and weight concerns.

If you think that this might be the case for you, we advise you to seek counseling or to talk to a close and trusted confidant who might help you explore these issues.

# YOUR PERSONALIZED PLAN

## Getting Started

In Chapter 37, The Guilt-Induced Stress-Eater's Cure, you will find simple, effective recommendations that are individualized specifically for the Guilt-Induced Stress-Eater. Read through Chapter 37 and apply the recommendations you find there to the Stress-Eating Cure Program (Chapters 21 through 29). These personalized suggestions will help turn the Stress-Eating Cure Program into your personalized Stress-Eating Cure.

## Special Note:

Guilt is a powerful emotion backed by a powerful hormone imbalance. Without the right tools, it can seem almost impossible to break free of guilt's grip.

Take time to read Chapter 37 and the Stress-Eating Cure Program carefully. Guilt-Induced Stress-Eaters are notorious for not taking care of themselves as well as they might take care of others. Consider how much care you might give to reading information that offers help for a problem that your friend, family member, or mate is having. Then give yourself twice as much time. After all, you've earned it!

# 18

# The Exhaustion-Induced Stress-Eater

Have you ever been so tired that you couldn't think? So exhausted that you hurt all over? Did you ever feel too tired to eat but found yourself grabbing anything to eat that was handy, barely bothering to chew it?

If these experiences have been rather rare occurrences, lasting only a short time, then you've had a taste of what Exhaustion-Induced Stress-Eaters live with on a full-time basis. On the other hand, if these experiences are part of your daily routine, you know that the experience of Exhaustion-Induced Stress-Eating can barely be described.

Exhaustion-Induced Stress-Eaters have described themselves as running on empty. Their minds and bodies have been pushed to the limit—beyond the limit—but they cannot or will not give up. They are both the heroes and the victims of today's world, yet those around them rarely understand or appreciate how hard they try and how great the cost.

*Exhaustion-Induced Stress-Eaters give too much,*
*too often, and far too well.*

On both a personal and professional note, we have rarely met an Exhaustion-Induced Stress-Eater we didn't like. They are the caretakers, givers, and doers; they rarely take the easy road and only under impossible duress do they ever give up.

That single-minded tenacity, however, is often their downfall. For, although they spend their time and energy meeting the demands of the moment, the needs of others, and the situation, they take almost no time to attend to their own needs for nourishment, rest, relaxation, and rejuvenation.

*Your proclamations of weariness are, most likely, cries for help.*

The words that Exhaustion-Induced Stress-Eaters speak can reveal the emotional and physical crises they face. "I'm at the end of my rope," some may say. "I can't keep going like this." "If I don't get some rest, I feel like I'm going to die!"

To others, their words may seem like exaggerations. Indeed, one of the most central problems is that Exhaustion-Induced Stress-Eaters themselves do not view the depths of their weariness with serious concern. In our experience, their thoughts and words of desperation barely reflect the levels of emotional and physical exhaustion these stress-eaters are experiencing.

As revealing as their words are, the tone with which they are said often conveys more. At first, an Exhaustion-Induced Stress-Eater may utter statements of upset only in response to uniquely frustrating events in a loud and clearly distraught voice. Upon coming home from work, for example, and finding that her son has turned the kitchen into a complete disaster area is enough to make any Exhaustion-Induced Stress-Eater mother shout, "I can't stand this anymore!"

*The less the emotion, the greater the exhaustion.*

As Exhaustion-Induced Stress-Eaters become more emotionally or physically depleted, however, the loudness and fury are likely to be replaced with far milder responses. Reactions to disappointments or frustrating experiences are likely to be spoken in a soft voice, lacking emotion, and seeming to carry a fair share of resignation.

A wife attempts to communicate with her husband. She discovers that, for what seems like the thousandth time, she is unable to make him understand. She may sigh and appear to give up.

"I can't do this anymore," she says softly. "I just don't have the strength."

Though her tone is filled with neither anger nor reproach, it would be a mistake to think this woman is no longer upset. She is, in fact, experiencing a hormonal backlash that overwhelms her and makes her virtually unable to respond.

The low adrenaline levels that characterize an Exhaustion-Induced Stress-Eater carry a hormonal history that, in many ways, echoes the emotional challenges an Exhaustion-Induced Stress-Eater has faced. In this Stress-Eating Pattern, adrenaline levels drop by a process of feedback that takes place when the body has been too stressed for too long.

Although adrenaline levels and other hormones might have surged through the bloodstream at one time, urging the stress-eater to take charge and make change, when adrenaline levels remain high for too long, the body begins to shut off and shut down to this hormone's impact.

Doorways into cells (receptor sites) close and start to disappear. At first the adrenal glands continue to pour adrenaline into the bloodstream, but as the levels continue to grow, the adrenals begin to cease their outpouring.

*Chances are, it's not just
your mind that's exhausted.*

The Exhaustion-Induced Stress-Eater has become adrenaline resistant and is suffering from adrenal fatigue,[1] the body's attempt to stop the onslaught of this hormone.

With high levels of insulin (from the frequent intake of carbohydrate-rich foods) stressing the body beyond it normal limitations, adrenaline levels in the bloodstream drop. The Exhaustion-Induced Stress-Eater's ability to take action and fight the stresses that threaten to overwhelm is disabled.

When Exhaustion-Induced Stress-Eaters say they have reached the end of their ropes, when they conclude that they are "burned out," they are, quite accurately, reflecting the depleted hormonal landscape that lies within.

---

[1] *There are many causes of adrenal fatigue. Only an appropriate health care professional can diagnose and recommend appropriate treatment for this condition.*

# YOUR PERSONALIZED PLAN

## Special Note:

If your Exhaustion-Induced Stress-Eating may be related to lack of sleep, take whatever steps are appropriate, well advised, and needed to immediately remedy the situation. No recommendation or eating plan can take the place of adequate sleep. Before you proceed, be sure that a lack of sleep is not at the core of your Exhaustion-Induced Stress-Eating. If you still meet the criteria of this Stress-Eating Pattern after getting adequate sleep, only then should you consider getting started on the program.

## GETTING STARTED

In Chapter 38, The Exhaustion-Induced Stress-Eater's Cure, you will find simple, effective recommendations that are individualized specifically for the Exhaustion-Induced Stress-Eater. Read through Chapter 38 and apply the recommendations you find there to the Stress-Eating Program (Chapters 21 through 29). These personalized suggestions will help turn the Stress-Eating Cure Program into your personalized Stress-Eating Cure.

# 19

# The Quicky
# Stress-Eater

Imagine life moving at a fast-forward speed. Words fade into gibberish, movements around you appear jerky and bizarre, and the emotions of others seem strangely distant. Welcome to the world of the Quicky Stress-Eater!

Quicky Stress-Eaters are in a class all their own. They have hormone levels that mark them as both stress-eaters *and* non-stress-eaters at the same time.

When they eat while under time constraints, Quicky Stress-Eaters can experience adrenaline levels far above the norm. Often, they grab what they can, eat on the run, bolt down their food, and barely taste what they are eating. During those rare times when they are not on the run—though they may still tend to eat quickly—their adrenaline levels remain within a normal range.

*Some eat on the run; some gulp and run.*

When they are pressured by time demands, Quicky Stress-Eaters can gulp down a meal and barely notice they have eaten. They often get little pleasure from their food. In many cases, Quicky Stress-Eaters eat because they must to minimize stress-hunger and cravings. They may experience a fleeting sense of relief with the first hurried bite, but when they've finished, a feeling of satisfaction eludes them.

High levels of adrenaline are the mainstay of the Quicky Stress-Eater and are known to keep oxytocin levels low. Oxytocin, the bonding hormone, opens you to intimate connections with others. The Quicky Stress-Eater, low in oxytocin, is strongly task-oriented and has little interest in conversation that focuses on feelings rather than facts.

Even though you may not be genetically prone to overrelease any of several hormones, an extended period of time-crushing demands can throw even the hardiest of systems quite out of whack.

Quicky Stress-Eating acts as a springboard from which many can catapult into one of many full-fledged Stress-Eating Patterns. Those who do not have the genetic tendency toward hormonal imbalances and for whom time demands are short-lived or who take control of the situation are likely to remain stress-eating free.

For those who do not or cannot avoid the powerful pull of Quicky Stress-Eating, however, this pattern can become what we might call Stress-Eating in Training.

The tipping point for the Quicky Stress-Eater appears to be the genetic predisposition of the potential stress-eater in combination with the duration of the demands. If you have a genetic tendency to release cortisol, insulin, or other hormones in great quantities, even a short period of demanding and urgent responsibilities can catapult you from Quicky Stress-Eating to any of the other Stress-Eating Patterns.

## YOUR PERSONALIZED PLAN

Your first task is going to be the hardest: As hard as it may be, you'll need to make time to read through the Stress-Eating Cure Program (Chapters 21 through 29) and your Personalized Plan in The Quicky Stress-Eater's Cure (Chapter 39). Then put them into action.

Once you begin to bring your adrenaline back into balance, the program will become an easy part of your routine. But first, you need to make the time to put you first!

## GETTING STARTED

In Chapter 39, you will find simple, effective recommendations individualized specifically for the Quicky Stress-Eater. Apply these recommendations to the Stress-Eating Cure Program (Chapters 21 through 29). These personalized suggestions will help turn the Stress-Eating Cure Program into your personalized Stress-Eating Cure.

# 20

# The Delayed
# Stress-Eater

Let's say you've experienced a stressful event that on a scale from one to ten qualified as about an eight. It might have been a health-related scare that turned out okay, a financial blow, or an argument with your spouse or teenage child. In the midst of the crisis, you found you had little desire to eat. Although the situation may have continued for a couple of days, your appetite remained almost nonexistent.

Then, imagine that the oddest thing happened: When the crisis passed, your appetite suddenly returned . . . with a vengeance. Although you were no longer in the midst of a stress-filled experience, you could not seem to stop eating.

The question, then, is: When is stress-eating not stress-eating?

Answer: When it is Delayed Stress-Eating.

Delayed Stress-Eating is experienced as the onset of stress-hunger and cravings after a stressful event has been resolved or stressful emotions have subsided. The high levels of cortisol that are released during moments of great stress lead to an intense hunger for any of a wide variety of foods. A strong desire for starches, snack food, junk food, sweets, or high-fat foods is typical. In addition, unusually strong cravings for specific foods, including pickles, pizza, Chinese food, chocolate, ice cream, milk, fried chicken, and salty, crunchy, or spicy foods, may be experienced as well.

*Hungry after the stress has passed?*
*That's your body, trying to get back to normal.*

Delayed Stress-Eating is not a Stress-Eating Pattern per se. In contrast to the overreactive response to stress that is the hallmark of

Stress-Eating Patterns, Delayed Stress-Eating is the natural, healthy, and proper response to a threat, fear, surprise, or any of a thousand challenges you may face.

At the greatest moments of stress, if all is in balance, hormones signal your body to conserve energy. The energy that would usually be allotted for the purposes of digestion and sex is channeled into the muscles, nerves, and organs needed to maintain the body at peak alertness and readiness.

Cortisol causes a rise in insulin and ghrelin, two powerful hormones that regulate hunger and cravings. These two metabolic regulators tell your body that it must have food. You experience an intense and immediate need to eat.

As insulin and ghrelin are rising, cortisol signals a decrease in serotonin and leptin, two hormones of satisfaction and weight-loss regulation. When levels of these two hormones fall too quickly or too low, you do not get the signal to stop eating. At the same time, your body is less able to burn the excess food you take in and is instead more likely to store it away in your fat cells.

When things go right, these processes are self-limiting. That is, they go on for a short time, then stop on their own. When cortisol levels remain too high for too long, however, they can become a prolonged, intractable self-reinforcing pattern.

*The good news:*
*In Delayed Stress-Eating,*
*excess is the exception, not the norm.*

## YOUR PERSONALIZED PLAN

Some Delayed Stress-Eaters will find they have no need for the Stress-Eating Cure Program. For others, the program will help them remain balanced and free from stress-eating for life.

Chapter 40, The Delayed Stress-Eater's Cure, will help guide you in which is the most appropriate and useful choice for you.

# GETTING STARTED

In Chapter 40 you will find simple, effective recommendations that are individualized specifically for the Delayed Stress-Eater. Read through Chapter 40 and, if the program seems appropriate for you, apply the recommendations you find there to the Stress-Eating Cure Program (Chapters 21 through 29). These personalized suggestions will help turn the Stress-Eating Cure Program into your personalized Stress-Eating Cure.

# PART
# IV

# 21

# Read This First:
# The Stress-Eating
# Cure Program

## BEFORE YOU BEGIN

Before you begin to learn about the program, please turn to the Contents and look over the titles on Chapters 30 through 40 (pages x–xi). Turn to the chapter that describes the cure for your Primary Stress-Eating Pattern and read the personalized recommendations offered there.

These recommendations may help you determine which plan is best for you (the Step-by-Step Plan versus the Quick-Start Plan). In addition, these recommendations may help in choosing the best Balancing Foods and Comfort Foods, as well as the most appropriate Stress-Eating Busters for your particular Stress-Eating Pattern.

After you have familiarized yourself with the recommendations appropriate to your Primary Stress-Eating Pattern, return to this page and get ready to begin.

You are about to discover the many pleasures and rewards of the Stress-Eating Cure, a revolutionary program specifically designed to put an end to stress-hunger, cravings, stress-eating, and the weight problems that result.

The Stress-Eating Cure Program includes:

1) Two eating programs from which you will choose. Each is designed to bring the body back into balance.

    A) The Step-by-Step Plan: a simple, one-change-at-a-time, comfortably paced eating plan

or

    B) The Quick-Start Plan: faster-paced eating changes that transform your eating in a matter of days

2) Stress-Eating Busters:

    Tips, strategies, and actions to further enhance hormonal balance and eliminate stress-eating and the weight problems that follow.

The aim of the Stress-Eating Cure Program is simple: to put an end to the stress-hunger, cravings, stress-eating, and weight problems that can run (and ruin) your life. After you realize that your stress-hunger, cravings, stress-eating, and weight problems spring from one or more of a variety of hormonal imbalances, you are halfway to success.

The other half comes from a program that will help you correct the hormonal imbalance that has been in control of your eating and your weight for far too long. And that program, of course, you hold right in hands.

This program is unlike any other you have ever experienced. Here are some surprising differences you can look forward to:

**This program does *not* require willpower.**

It has been designed to correct the *physical* cause of your stress-hunger, cravings, stress-eating, and weight problems.

**You can enjoy your favorite foods—every day— without weighing or measuring them.**

As you follow the program, you will no longer feel an overwhelming *need* to overeat or to eat too often.

**Your weight loss should be steady, without the frustration of weight-loss plateaus.**

As the hormones that regulate your fat storage and weight loss begin to normalize, excess weight will drop steadily and without struggle.

**Your confidence, energy, motivation, and outlook on life will improve easily, naturally.**

As the stress-hunger, cravings, stress-eating, and pounds slip away, you may rediscover feelings of hope and happiness that you forgot were even there.

To reap these benefits, and a whole lot more, here's what we suggest:

1) Read through the program that follows, from start to finish. Please don't skim and expect to understand the plan. You're almost sure to miss vital points required to assure your success. This program has been designed to help bring you the life you want and deserve. It deserves at least as much of your attention as you would give to a good novel. After all, as they say, you're worth it!

2) After you have read through the program, begin the program only when you feel ready. You might find that it makes sense to start when you have a little time off from work and can focus on the changes you want to make. Some people find that a vacation is the perfect time to begin!

As odd as it sounds at first, consider this: Vacation time means a break from the routine; hopefully a bit more time for yourself; and, best of all, if you will be traveling and dining in restaurants, you will have a wide variety of choices (not limited by time preparation considerations as you would at home). As an added boost, someone else will be doing the cooking. These two luxuries can add a new twist of adventure and fun to your new program and offer you options you might not have considered at home. Since you will be enjoying the food you love every day, you need not worry about sacrificing the pleasure of wonderful meals while away. As an added bonus, imagine how delightful it would be to enjoy yourself fully on vacation and return having lost weight!

If you spend vacation time at home or cook for yourself while away, starting the program at that time will allow you to focus your needs without the usual demands of daily life.

3) There is a wonderful saying that advises, "Take what you need and leave the rest." Although this program works as a whole and should not be mixed and matched with diets from your past, if the guidelines or suggestions you find in these pages are not right for *you* or are not right *at this time*, don't push yourself to follow them. As in all things, use your own judgment as well as that of your physician.

Guidelines and suggestions are simply that: recommendations as to what *should, could,* or *will most likely* work. If it's not right for you or if you simply don't want to do it, by all means, don't!

With that said, it's time to choose an eating plan and get started!

## STEP-BY-STEP VERSUS QUICK-START: WHICH DO I CHOOSE?

The Step-by-Step Plan guides you in making seven small changes, one at a time, over a period of 2 weeks.

Each progressive change (called a *step*) builds on the steps that have come before. Each is made easier by the skills acquired and the hormonal balance achieved at the previous step.

Each step contains a guideline that details the simple change that should be made at that step. Guidelines will direct you to add, balance, or delay the eating of certain foods at certain meals.

*You will never be asked to give up the foods you love or be required to limit yourself to small portions.*

Each day, you will enjoy a Big Balanced Breakfast or an Alternative Meal,[1] in which you can enjoy your favorite foods along with other foods that will help balance your hormonal response.

---

[1] The Alternative Meal is a daily, balanced meal that replaces the Big Balanced Breakfast. It may be eaten at any time later in the day or evening. In combination with Balancing Foods (pages 244–47), it should always contain a good portion of Comfort Foods (pages 248–51).

With each change, as the physical cause of your stress-eating is reduced, then eliminated, you will gain greater control over your eating and you will begin to lose weight almost without trying.

As you complete Step #6 of the Step-by-Step Plan, you will have the eating portion of the Stress-Eating Cure Program firmly in hand.

On the Quick-Start Plan, you will make the same changes to your eating routine, but the changes will take place within a matter of 2 or 3 days.

*Same destination,*
*different time frames.*

Both the Quick-Start Plan and the Step-by-Step Plan take you to the same end point eating-wise; they differ only in how quickly you will get there and how many changes you make at once.

On the Quick-Start Plan, you may begin to notice a significant decrease in stress-hunger and cravings by the 2nd or 3rd day. The pounds should begin to fall away at the same time.

On the Step-by-Step Plan, you will have incorporated the same changes, but with complete ease and at a more comfortable pace!

At the end of 12 days on the Step-by-Step Plan, you can expect the same elimination of stress-hunger, cravings, and stress-eating, as well as the same weight loss as those who have chosen to move at a quicker pace.

In both plans, as you incorporate eating changes, you will be offered a wide variety of Stress-Eating Busters, tips, strategies, and actions you can take to further ensure your hormonal balance and eliminate or greatly reduce the impact of future stressors.

**REMEMBER:** Whether you choose the Step-by-Step Plan or the Quick-Start Plan, at the end of 12 days, you will be following the same program. The only difference is how many changes you make at once and how quickly you make them.

If you would like a smooth, easy transition, one that you'll barely notice, choose the Step-by-Step Plan and move one step at a time. If you want immediate results, try the Quick-Start Plan.

The good news is that your choice is not written in stone. You may start off with the Step-by-Step Plan and realize that the changes you're making are so easy that you'd have no problem moving at a much faster pace. If so, you have two choices.

You can feel free to move more quickly through the Step-by-Step Plan, adding one or two changes each day. Or, if you prefer, move to the Quick-Start Plan and make all the changes at once.

On the other hand, if at first you think that the Quick-Start Plan is more your style but, after a day or two, decide that you would prefer to take things a bit more slowly, simply take a step sideways, and start again with the Step-by-Step Plan.

# STARTING POINTS

Both of the eating plans of the Stress-Eating Cure Program begin by making changes to your *normal or usual* way of eating. For the purposes of the program, this is your *starting point*. Your starting point, however, is unlike that of anyone else.

In recent weeks, you may have been stress-eating throughout the day, at every meal and snack. Or, maybe you've been attempting to stick to a weight-loss regimen or a generally healthy eating plan, only to find yourself slipping or *cheating* when the cravings or life's stresses become too great. You may have been holding on by pure willpower to the pounds you've lost on any of a number of programs, knowing that it was only a matter of time before you gained it all back.

It doesn't matter how you got to here; we're just glad that you did. The Stress-Eating Cure Program will help transform any starting point into a turning point.

If, for example, you have been eating carbohydrate-rich foods throughout the day, the guidelines at each step will guide you in the addition of a variety of foods that will help balance your hormones, break the craving cycle, and quickly get you back in control.

If you have had only occasional lapses into stress-eating, each of the guidelines will help you to achieve the consistency that is essential in maintaining hormonal balance, keeping stress-hunger, cravings, and stress-eating from returning, achieving a steady weight loss, and ulti-mately maintaining that weight loss without struggle.

The Sample Menus that follow in each of the six steps of the pro-gram are based on the assumption that, as you begin this plan, your stress-eating is in high gear and that you may be eating carbohydrate-rich, high-fat foods throughout the day (in meals and/or snacks).

If this assumption is accurate, the menus will offer guidance on how to progress through each of the six guidelines that follow.

Of course, there's the possibility that, as you start this program, you are *not* caught in a Stress-Eating Cycle and that you are *not* consuming carbohydrate-rich and/or high-fat foods (Comfort Foods) more than two or three times a day. If this is the case, do *not* increase your intake of Comfort Foods to match the Sample Menus shown. Simply use each guideline to make desired changes to your eating as it was when you came to this program.

In any case, you're in for an adventure. We know! We've been there and, happily, we discovered an incredibly easy and rewarding way out. Now, we're here to help you.

A new way of life lies before you, a whole new start, a new way to conquer an old foe that has haunted you for far too long. And we'll be there with you every step of the way.

It's time to get started!

To begin either the Step-by-Step Plan or the Quick-Start Plan, go to Chapter 22. From there, you'll be guided to the right path for you.

# 22

# The Quick-Start Plan

The Quick-Start and Step-by-Step Plans are identical programs with one exception: The Step-by-Step Plan requires 12 days to incorporate all of the guidelines into your life. On the Quick-Start Plan, you will accomplish the same feat within 3 to 4 days.

*Important Note:* Before deciding which plan best suits your needs, read through Chapter 21. The information you find there will give you a better understanding of the pros and cons of each of the plans, and it contains essential information on the program as well.

## GETTING STARTED

Assuming that it's advisable and appropriate for you to move at a more advanced rate, here's the best way to proceed on the Quick-Start Plan.

1. Carefully read Chapters 23 and 24. These chapters contain information that is important to your success on the program along with the guideline for Step #1, the addition of a Big Balanced Breakfast or Alternative Meal[1] to your usual meals and snacks.

   Step #1 calls for 2 days of practice if you are on the Step-by-Step Plan. If you are on the Quick-Start Plan, however, this guideline should be considered fulfilled when you have successfully incorporated it for 1 day.

   *Note:* If it takes more than 1 day to get *any* step right, take an extra day or two so that you can do it with ease.

---

[1] The Alternative Meal is a daily balanced meal that replaces the Big Balanced Breakfast. It may be eaten at any time later in the day or evening. In combination with Balancing Foods (pages 244–47), it should always contain a good portion of Comfort Foods (pages 248–51).

2. When you have added a Big Balanced Breakfast or Alternative Meal to your eating program for 1 day without any difficulties, you are ready to move to the next steps.

3. Read over both Steps #2 and #3 (Chapters 25 and 26) before incorporating the next guideline(s). After reading both chapters, incorporate guidelines from these two chapters *at the same time*; that is, include Balancing Proteins in all meals and snacks as indicated and, at the same time, include Balancing Vegetables and Salad in all meals (with the exception of Big Balanced Breakfasts or your usual breakfast).

   Although Steps #2 and #3 call for 2 days of practice each, on the Quick-Start Plan, these guidelines will be considered met when you have successfully incorporated them at the same time for 1 day.

4. Go directly to Step #6.

   *Please note:* We are fully aware that, on the Quick-Start Plan, you are leapfrogging the intermediate steps of the Step-by-Step Plan. By meeting the guideline of a more advanced step, however, you will automatically meet the guidelines of all the steps that came before.

5. Read Chapter 29, Step #6, and incorporate this step's guideline into your eating program (while still following the guidelines from Steps #1, #2, and #3).

   You may be able to add the guideline from Step #6 in 1 day, or it may take a few days of practice to get it comfortably in place.

To make your program run more smoothly, we suggest that you plan your meals and snacks the previous day. If all goes well, you'll have learned what works. If it doesn't, you'll know what needs to be worked out, and you can plan better for the following day.

If you hit some glitches while trying to incorporate Step #6 into your life all at once, take a couple of steps backward, literally. Go to Step #4, then move forward one step at a time.

Should you still not be able to meet the guidelines of Step #4, we strongly suggest that you start back at Step #1 and work your way through the program from the beginning, giving yourself at least 2 days to get it right at each step. Sometimes the fastest way through is by taking things at a slower, but steadier pace.

As you put Step #6 into action, either immediately or by taking it a bit more slowly, read through Chapter 41 and incorporate the Stress-Eating Busters that you find there into your daily life.

When you have the final step in place, you will find yourself at the beginning of a whole new journey of freedom, choice, and balance of mind, body, and spirit. It's a remarkable adventure.

# 23

# The Big Breakfast Breakthrough

## DON'T WANT A BIG BREAKFAST? NO TIME? NO WORRIES!

If you simply cannot or prefer not to eat a Big Balanced Breakfast, you can still reap the benefits of this program!

Read through this chapter first. The information you find here may surprise you.

If you still prefer to pass on the Big Balanced Breakfast, either in general or on occasion, we have a simple solution.

In Chapter 24 you will discover the perfect substitute to the Big Balanced Breakfast: an Alternative Meal that can be enjoyed as you desire, any time later in the day or evening.

## WHY A BIG BREAKFAST?

When it comes to those who are stress-eaters, there is one thing that you can pretty much count on: They skip breakfast on a regular basis.

The simple rule of thumb is: Show us a stress-eater and we can almost certainly show you someone who doesn't start the day with a good meal.

Some stress-eaters simply have no desire to eat in the morning; others just don't have the time; many harbor the erroneous belief that the calories they save in the morning are better spent on meals and snacks they eat later in the day.

"Why should I eat breakfast when I'm not hungry?" they reason. "I'll only get hungry later and want to eat again."

Their logic is right! In reality, however, it doesn't quite work like that. The less you eat at breakfast, the more you eat as the day goes on. Eating a Big Balanced Breakfast turns out to be the best use of calories.

*Now, you are eating for four!*
*And they are all hormones.*

Even more to the point, on this program, eating a Big Balanced Breakfast is not aimed at satisfying your early morning hunger. We know that you may not feel like eating until later in the day. For the purpose of cutting cravings, stress-hunger, stress-eating, and weight gain, a good breakfast helps balance your hormone levels when you need it the most.

With each dawn, your body shifts into high gear and readies you to go out and hunt for food. Not knowing that your most challenging battle is likely to be getting the kids off to school or making it to work on time, your cortisol, adrenaline, and insulin levels reach their highest points of the day. Other hormones join the rising tide and await the food that will end the fast your body has endured all night.

As you wash and dress, your nerves and muscles virtually vibrate in anticipation. All has been made ready for the incoming feast. You head toward the kitchen, and your adrenaline and cortisol rise even higher. Oxytocin levels fall; the only need for bonding your body has right now is the bonding it desires with some good, satisfying food.

You're at the kitchen now, and your body is in perfect readiness . . . except that you bypass that room and head for the door. You're off to work before your body knows what has happened. You'll get something on the way to the office, you tell yourself. Or, you conclude, you just don't have the inclination or the time (or both) for breakfast.

On the other hand, you might have stopped at the kitchen and paid a small and hurried tribute to your nutritional (and hormonal) needs. A quick cup of coffee and some toast or a bagel or some cold cereal. You tell yourself that you've done your duty, and you're ready to take on the day.

*A little breakfast can be far worse
than a big balanced one.*

In effect, however, you've done more damage than good. With just a bit of, but not enough, high-carb food to start your day, you've spiked your insulin levels even higher. Within a short time, your blood sugar levels may begin to fluctuate madly, with cortisol and adrenaline levels echoing the hormonal chaos.

It's no wonder that, later in the day, when you do start eating, you are barely able to stop. You have been attempting to hold back the hormonal floodgates, and you are almost certain to be swept away by the ensuing torrent.

Naturally slim people instinctively balance their morning hormone surplus. They eat breakfast, bring their hormones back into balance, and move on to the rest of their day. Those who are overweight and overweight stress-eaters, in particular, get caught up in an early morning hormone overload from which it is hard to break free. Few ever realize that it may well be what they *didn't* eat that may be driving their stress-eating for the rest of the day.

Here's what scientists have discovered about the breakfast-obesity connection.

As they later reported in the *American Journal of Epidemiology*, researchers at the University of Massachusetts Medical School studied the eating habits of hundreds of people over the course of a year. Taking into consideration the many behaviors that can contribute to excess weight, these scientists concluded that "skipping breakfast was associated with an increased prevalence of obesity."

Using data from the National Health and Nutrition Examination Survey on more than 16,000 individuals, scientists concluded that "skipping breakfast is not an effective way to manage weight." Reporting on the findings of supportive studies by fellow researchers, they also noted that "breakfast eaters tend to have a lower body mass index than breakfast skippers, and obese individuals are more likely to skip breakfast or consume less energy at breakfast."

*Eat before noon, lose the weight soon.*
*Eat in the night, regret the first bite.*

Of great interest were the findings that Night-Eating Syndrome is characterized, in part, by habitual breakfast skipping and that "moderately obese women lost more weight when they consumed 70 percent of their daily intake before noon instead of in the afternoon and evening."

The final report these scientists offered was of particular interest to anyone who has ever doubted how important breakfast is in a weight-loss program. "Lean individuals," they concluded, "lose weight when consuming a 2,000-calorie meal at breakfast but tend to gain weight if the meal was eaten at dinner." While we are, most certainly, *not* recommending a 2,000-calorie breakfast in addition to a day's worth of other foods, it is interesting to note that the same food eaten at either breakfast or dinner can result in weight loss versus weight gain.

In two of the many other studies reporting similar findings, scientists reporting in the *Journal of the American College of Nutrition* observed that overweight subjects consume a less-varied breakfast, spend less time eating breakfast, and consume smaller quantities of food than do normal-weight subjects. A team of scientists from research facilities throughout the United Kingdom studied more than 6,000 men and women and confirmed that the less energy consumed at breakfast, the greater the weight gain. Their recommendation: "Redistribution of daily energy intake, so that more energy is consumed at breakfast and less energy is consumed later in the day, may help to reduce weight gain in middle-aged adults."

Other studies have reported similar findings and offered similar solutions for overweight children, adolescents, and adults of all ages.

In a study of 6,764 middle-aged men and women, these researchers found that the larger the breakfast, the less snacking in the evening.
Purslow et al., *American Journal of Epidemiology,* 2007

Subjects who skipped breakfast three or more times per week showed significant greater likelihood of Night-Eating Syndrome, binge-eating, and obesity.

> Colles et al., *International Journal of Obesity*, 2007

After full, carbohydrate-rich mixed breakfasts, subjects experienced a 40 percent increase in alertness, showed a 36 percent long-term decrease in hunger through to lunch, and consumed 75 percent less food throughout the day, as compared to those who ate a more modest, protein-rich breakfast.

> Holt et al., *International Journal of Food Sciences and Nutrition*, 2009

Those who consumed more frequent meals, particularly breakfast, and snacks weighed less.

Eating more frequently, having breakfast, and consuming three meals every day have potentially important clinical applications for the treatment of Binge-Eating Disorder.

> Masheb et al., *Behavioral Research Therapy*, 2006

As breakfasts decreased, snacks increased.

> Rolland-Cachera et al., *International Journal of Obesity-Related Metabolic Disorders*, 2004

Large, mixed breakfasts resulted in significantly higher satiety scores, reduced hunger, and 50 percent lower rates of fatigue.

> Pasman, *International Journal of Obesity*, 2003

Those who skip breakfast have 4.5 times increased odds for obesity compared with those who eat breakfast regularly.

Eating a healthy breakfast is associated with energy balance and weight control.

> Greenwood et al., *Journal of the American Board of Family Medicine*, 2008

Eating breakfast helps sustain weight loss.

An ongoing study by the National Weight Control Registry of individuals who lost 30 or more pounds and kept it off for at least 1 year found that 78 percent of the nearly 3,000 participants ate breakfast every day.
     Sitzman, *American Association of Human Nutrition*, 2006

In a study of 2,959 subjects, these researchers concluded that "eating breakfast is a characteristic common to successful weight loss maintainers."
     Wyatt et al., *Obesity Research*, 2002

Of greatest importance to the stress-eater, however, was discovery of the hormone connection to big breakfasts and weight loss.

The results showed that stress was associated with higher cortisol levels, and daily consumption of breakfast cereal was associated with lower cortisol levels.
     Smith, *Nutritional Neuroscience*, 2002

Omitting breakfast impairs fasting lipids and postprandial insulin sensitivity and could lead to weight gain.
     Hamid et al., *American Journal of Clinical Nutrition*, 2005

All of these remarkable scientific findings might have remained in the realm of the theoretical had it not been for one study that put these observations to work for those who need it most.

In 2008, two independent research teams on two different continents, working in tandem, revealed an extraordinary discovery: A research weight-loss regimen that included a big, well-balanced breakfast led to a fivefold increase in weight loss.

At the Endocrine Society's annual meeting in 2008, Dr. Daniela Jakubowicz and colleagues reported that at 32 weeks, big breakfast dieters (who included a balance of carbohydrate-rich foods in their early morning meal) lost 21.3 percent of their baseline weight as compared with a

4.5 percent decrease seen in those on a lower-calorie, low-carbohydrate diet (40 pounds versus 9 pounds).

As part of their weight-loss diet, subjects who consumed a big breakfast (including a balance of carbohydrate-rich foods at that meal) showed a significant decrease in hunger, increase in satiety, decreased desire to eat, and increased fullness.

"In the morning, the body is primed with hormones like adrenaline and cortisol and ready with the 'machinery' to convert protein to energy," Dr. Jakubowicz said. "The carbohydrates and protein also give a greater sense of satiety in the morning.

"A diet consisting of a high carbohydrate and protein breakfast facilitates weight loss by reducing hunger and diminishing carbohydrate craving."

Not only did a big breakfast lead to dramatically greater weight-loss outcomes, but it also resulted in far greater satisfaction, significantly less hunger, and freedom from carbohydrate cravings as well. Of greatest importance, however, was the fact that, in her reports of her research findings, Dr. Jakubowicz linked stress hormones to the remarkable impact that a big breakfast had on weight loss.

Within days of the research report, TV news, newspapers, and the Internet echoed an astounding response. Only 1 week after the unheralded release of the study's findings, more than 50,000 Web sites, blogs, and international media outlets were reporting the big breakfast breakthrough news and its apparent stress-hormone connection. Here's just a sampling.

# Big, Well-Balanced Breakfast Aids Weight Loss

*Reuters Health News*

### Summary:

Research subjects who included a big breakfast in their diet plans:

- Lost five times the weight, compared to those on a restrictive diet
- Lost 40 pounds versus 9 pounds
- Had significantly less hunger
- Experienced fewer carbohydrate cravings

# "Big Breakfast" Dieters Shed Pounds: Study Shows Big Breakfast Reduces Food Cravings Later in the Day

*WebMD News*

### Summary:

Research reveals that subjects on a diet that included a big breakfast:

- Lost 21 percent of their body weight
- Continued to lose weight for the full 8 months of the study (compared to those on restrictive diets who regained weight)
- Had significantly less hunger and fewer carbohydrate cravings

The American Dietetic Association says these "findings make perfect sense."

# Carb-Loading at Breakfast Makes Dieting Easier Long-Term

*MedpageToday.com*

### Summary:

Research indicates that a big breakfast as part of the diet significantly:

- Reduced cravings overall
- Reduced cravings for sweets, carbohydrates, starches, and fast food
- Decreased hunger
- Increased satiety
- Increased the sense of fullness, which lasted until 11:00 p.m.

# Early Morning Feasts Are the Secret to Beating Middle-Age Spread

*Mailonline News Service, United Kingdom*

### Summary:

Based on a 5-year study of nearly 7,000 subjects at Addenbrooke's Hospital in Cambridge, researchers concluded:

- Big breakfasters ate more in the morning, less in the evening, and weighed significantly less.
- "Breakfast like a king, dinner like a pauper" is especially true in middle age.
- Whether or not breakfast is skipped may affect weight gain more than how much food is eaten throughout the day.
- Skipping breakfast may prompt the body to store lunch and dinner as fat.
- Eating 50 percent of daily calories at breakfast gives the body time to metabolize calories more efficiently.
- The National Obesity Forum agrees: "Starting the day with a good breakfast is a good way to tackle weight gain."

## GETTING STARTED

In Step #1 (the chapter that follows), you'll discover the first guideline to get you started on your new adventure. You'll also find answers to the following questions and more.

When it comes to a Big Balanced Breakfast:

What foods should I include?

What foods *can't* I have?

How big should the breakfast be?

What do you mean by *balanced*?

What time should I eat my Big Balanced Breakfast?

What can I do if I don't have any time for breakfast?

Suppose I just don't want breakfast?

Take a breath and turn the page. You're about to learn everything you need to get started. We'll be with you every step of the way.

# 24

# Step #1:
# Cutting Cravings

## GUIDELINE:

### Begin each day with a Big Balanced Breakfast (or, if desired, enjoy an Alternative Meal later in the day or evening).

While adding this guideline, continue to eat your usual meals and snacks at all other times.

The importance of a Big Balanced Breakfast is no longer debated. As you discovered in Chapter 23, scientists have confirmed that if you want to get slim, stay healthy, balance your hormones, and stop stress-eating, a Big Balanced Breakfast is the way to go.

For non-breakfast eaters, however, there is another choice: the Alternative Meal. If you're *not* a willing big breakfast eater, you'll still get to have your cake and eat it too, so to speak. You'll just get to eat it later in the day or evening. Details follow!

## STEP #1 IN A NUTSHELL

1. In this first step of your program, you will be choosing from the list of Balancing Proteins (pages 244–46) and from the list of Comfort Foods (pages 248–51). Take a look at these lists now.

2. From this point on, start each day with a Big Balanced Breakfast or later in the day choose an Alternative Meal in its place.

3. In every Big Balanced Breakfast (or Alternative Meal), equal amounts of Balancing Proteins and Comfort Foods should be included (details and samples to come).

4. Take a day to try the Big Balanced Breakfast or Alternative Meal on for size, a second day to get comfortable with it.

   Move on to the next step if you have been able to add the Big Balanced Breakfast or Alternative Meal for 2 days without any difficulties.

   If there was a time when you didn't include the foods you wanted or when you weren't able to secure some uninterrupted time to enjoy them, if you found it difficult to fit into your schedule, or if you missed a Big Balanced Breakfast or Alternative Meal, continue at this step until you get it right for 2 full days.

   Don't linger at any one step too long. Consider what needs to be done to get the food you need and the time to enjoy it, then apply a little healthy selfishness on your own behalf.

5. As you are fulfilling this guideline, read through Chapter 41, Stress-Eating Busters. It's an important chapter. The information you will find there, especially related to Comfort Food Act-Alikes, can be essential to stopping your stress-hunger, cravings, and stress-eating immediately. The remaining Stress-Eating Busters can help keep you free of stress-eating in the face of future stresses and keep your weight-loss rate steady in the long term.

Now, to help you along the way, here are some of the most frequently asked questions and the answers you need to get started.

## What foods should I include in my Big Balanced Breakfast?

To fulfill the requirements of Step #1, you simply need to start each day with a breakfast that includes a healthy balance of foods. Include foods that are good for you along with foods that you enjoy the most.

In the best of worlds, these foods are the same, but as we all know only too well, those foods we enjoy the most are not always the ones that are best for us.

*Think about what you really want to eat!*
*This is your Big Balanced Breakfast. Make it worthwhile.*

As a general guide, of all the foods that are good for you, choose the ones you enjoy the most. If blueberry yogurt gives you delight and the thought of eggs turns your stomach, go for what pleases you! On the other hand, unless your health needs dictate otherwise, if you love a good omelet, enjoy your eggs without guilt.

This is your Big Balanced Breakfast—a special time each day when the world of food choice is open and welcoming. Your selections can include virtually any food you love (with the proviso that the food is not prohibited because of health concerns). You may choose from the long list of Balancing Foods (pages 244–47) in combination with our array of Comfort Foods (pages 248–51).

As an alternative, you may simply allow yourself to peruse the aisles of your supermarket. You may choose from the menu at your favorite restaurant or cook up a storm. The realm from which you will make your choices is limited only by your imagination.

We urge you, then, to not limit yourself to those dishes that are generally considered to be "breakfast" foods. We have never understood why some foods are considered breakfast foods and others are not.

We have often wondered why it is perfectly acceptable to have a slice of ham with your eggs, for example, but unusual to have a pork chop; why is sausage okay, but a hot dog seems strange? Many people love smoked or poached salmon but would frown at the thought of tuna salad. It seems particularly odd to us that it's acceptable to have steak and eggs at a brunch, but rarely do most folks think of steak, by itself, as a breakfast food (unless you were a cowboy in the old West).

*You have the whole wide world to choose from.*
*You don't have to limit yourself to breakfast foods!*

On a personal note, we love warm chicken salad for breakfast or cold pizza. When we're at home, we include a variety of different flavors; chicken, beef, pork, lamb, tuna salad, eggs, and cheese are all part of our typical homemade smorgasbord.

When we cook at home, we make several extra servings and pack them up in half-meal freezer bags. When needed, we take two out and heat them up in the microwave. We take out a half-serving of chicken with almonds and a half-serving of spicy shrimp stir-fry, add a yogurt and fruit sundae and some of our favorite chocolate cake for dessert, and voilà, instant feast!

You'll find sample meal plans later in this chapter but, for now, simply allow your mind to open to the world of possibilities that await you when you enjoy a Big Balanced Breakfast every day.

*What a trade-off! If you balance your food,*
*you get to eat the food you love the most!*

## What foods *can't* I have?

When it comes to this program, as long as you balance your breakfast, there are no foods that are off-limits to you at this meal. As in all matters, if your health care provider has told you to avoid or limit your intake of certain foods, that recommendation, of course, should be your prime directive.

With that consideration in mind, the wonderful array of Comfort Foods that you would enjoy both within and outside of a weight-reducing program is available to you at your Big Balanced Breakfast.

As you will discover in the next few pages, in this step you will combine your intake of Comfort Foods with Balancing Foods in order to help keep your hormone levels in balance.

This one requirement, that you balance your foods, is more easily fulfilled than you might imagine. You would like a stack of pancakes for breakfast? Fine, order some eggs, too, or a nice portion of breakfast meat on the side.

We would ask that you use some common sense, too. Your Big

Balanced Breakfast is not meant to be an excuse to binge. Choose a healthy variety of good foods that will supply you with the nutrition you need . . . but, at the same time, make sure they really hit the spot.

Before we move on, it's essential to address the subject of dietary fats. For health reasons and hormone balance as well, it's important to choose foods high in unsaturated fats. Avoid foods high in saturated fats and, most certainly, those containing trans fats. (See page 253 for a quick and simple guide to dietary fats.)

Finally, enjoy olive oil whenever you can! With the whole wide world of food choices available to you at your Big Balanced Breakfast, you can afford to make some smart, unsaturated fat selections for the good of your hormones, your heart, your weight, and your life.

## A Quick Word about Fast Foods

Although some of the foods you can buy at fast-food restaurants feel like the ultimate in Comfort Foods, in general, try to choose foods that are closer to nature. Minimally processed foods are better for you nutritionally and, at the same time, less likely to throw your hormonal balance off. Two scrambled eggs and ham made from the real thing are a far better choice than some unknown egg substitute and mystery meat sandwich. If you're going to have a special milk shake treat, try to make it with real milk and real ice cream. Unless otherwise advised, the closer to natural you can go, the better.

## What about sodas, power drinks, diet drinks, flavored waters, and such?

What you drink can make all the difference in the world! We have seen people break their Stress-Eating Patterns and lose a great deal of weight simply by giving up sugar substitutes.

The issue of what you *can* and *can't* have with regards to nonalcoholic beverages doesn't really become important until Step #4. We're going to hold off addressing the best choices in drinks until then.

For now, consider the following recommendation: A stress-eater's best choices are plain water, seltzer, sparkling water, tea (without any sweetener, that is, no sugar and no sugar substitute), or coffee (regular or decaffeinated, without any sweetener, that is, no sugar and no sugar substitute).

If you must have a sweetened drink or soda, sugar-sweetened drinks are better choices than those sweetened with any sugar substitute.

We know it's kind of strange to think of drinking sugar-sweetened drinks when you're used to sugar substitutes. Sugar seems to have less impact on your stress-hunger, cravings, stress-eating, and weight gain, however, than do sugar substitutes.

*Important Note:* Your individual health needs, blood sugar and glucose tolerance requirements, and physician's recommendations should always determine your choice of sweetener.

See Chapter 41 for essential information on Beverages and Comfort Food Act-Alikes, a more thorough look at the research, and alternative suggestions.

## What about alcoholic drinks?

Alcohol is in a class of its own. It is included in the Comfort Foods list because it can elicit similar hormonal imbalances as do sweets, starches, and other Comfort Foods. However, alcohol should *never* be considered a Comfort Food in the common use of the phrase.

Alcoholic drinks should be consumed *only when appropriate and safe* and always as part of a Big Balanced Breakfast or Alternative Meal. When alcohol is not clearly appropriate as part of a Big Balanced Breakfast, it can be included in an Alternative Meal and consumed later in the day or evening.

## How big should the Big Balanced Breakfast be? What size portions should I choose?

This is always a fun question to answer! Our response is usually: How big would you like it to be? If you are asking this question, it's pretty likely that you have endured more than your share of absurdly tiny meals, maddening portion control, and rigid and restrictive diets.

You won't find directives on how much (or how little) to eat on this program because as your hormones return to balance, you will choose adequate and appropriate portions—naturally.

The drive to consume great quantities of food is a *symptom* of the underlying disorder. When that disorder is corrected, the symptom will disappear.

Until the time you reach your hormonal balance—that is, during the short time that it will take for you to move through the six steps of the program—do *not* force yourself to eat less than you really want. Do make certain that you balance your Comfort Foods with Balancing Foods (as we will explain in the next few pages), but do not restrict your portions. Scientists have repeatedly reported that restrictive dieting in combination with stress and available food make up a triad of temptation that predictably leads to binge eating.

As your hormones find their ideal level, your stress-hunger, cravings, stress-eating, and weight concerns should become a thing of the past. Remember that slim, non-stress-eaters don't weigh and measure their food. Their bodies guide them in choosing just the right portions for maximum satisfaction. They do not need to control or limit themselves because they don't feel the impulse to overeat. As hard as it is to imagine, that is your goal as well.

## What do you mean by a *balanced* breakfast?

Imagine, for a moment, that you are standing in front of two large bags of pebbles; one is filled with black stones and the other with white stones. Now, consider that you are asked to reach in and take out equal fistfuls of pebbles, one color to each hand. Sounds easy, doesn't it? That's how simple it is to balance your Big Balanced Breakfast.

Each day, you will enjoy both Comfort Foods and Balancing Foods, in equal amounts, at your Big Balanced Breakfast or Alternative Meal. Comfort Foods are those foods that many people find most pleasurable. By no coincidence, they are also those foods that have been shown to strongly impact the stress-eater's hormonal balance.

## What are Comfort Foods?
## What are Balancing Foods?

Though they offer comfort and pleasure, when Comfort Foods are eaten without a good portion of Balancing Foods, they throw your body's hormonal equilibrium out of kilter. Comfort Foods give you comfort; Balancing Foods give you balance. Together, you can have it all.

Comfort Foods are often rich in carbohydrates and/or contain large quantities of saturated fat. The less-sweet and less-processed of these foods, such as grains, bread, fruit, potatoes, pasta, and rice, provide your body with the carbohydrates it needs to keep you healthy. All starchy vegetables, fruits, and fruit juices should be considered Comfort Foods as well.

Comfort Foods also include all sorts of desserts and snack foods such as potato chips, pretzels, cakes, pies, doughnuts, cookies, chocolate, ice cream, and other sugary treats. Comfort Foods also include any food or drink that contains sugar substitutes of any kind. If a food or drink *tastes* sweet, your body responds to it as if it contains sugar, releasing many of the same hormones that can increase your stress-hunger and cravings and lead to stress-eating and weight gain. At your daily Big Balanced Breakfast or Alternative Meal, Comfort Foods should be combined with equal amounts of Balancing Foods.

Balancing Foods (see pages 244–47), on the other hand, are those foods that help equalize your hormone levels. Essentially, they *balance out* the effects of Comfort Foods. Balancing Foods are usually low in carbohydrates, low in saturated fat, and, depending on the type of food, high in fiber. Balancing Foods include a wide variety of lean proteins (meat, fish, chicken, turkey, eggs, etc.) and low-carbohydrate, high-fiber vegetables (green beans, green pepper, mushrooms, cucumbers, etc.). Included under Balancing Foods are a wide variety of nuts and cheeses as well.

When Balancing Foods and Comfort Foods are eaten in combination, in approximately equal portions, they can provide you with the pleasure of the foods you greatly enjoy without the hormonal rebound that can drive you to stress-eat.

## What time should I eat my Big Balanced Breakfast?

One question, two answers: First, it's best to eat your Big Balanced Breakfast as early in your day as possible. Second, wait to eat your Big Balanced

Breakfast until you have a full variety of satisfying foods, divided equally between Comfort Foods and Balancing Foods. Ideally, this would also be a time when you are less likely to be interrupted and can concentrate on taking care of your own needs and enjoying yourself fully.

Imagine a typical workday. Let's assume that you consider grabbing a quick snack as you bolt out the door. You are not certain whether the eat-on-the-run choice at 7:30 a.m. is a better choice than the option of leaving home a bit early and calling ahead to the restaurant across the street from work. With the restaurant option, you could pick up a delicious meal and enjoy it at your desk before your workday begins. Your breakfast would not take place until 8:30 a.m., however.

In this case, choose the full meal at work. A later but satisfying breakfast takes precedence. Once you've picked up your meal and arrived at work, however, make certain that you do not delay in getting to your meal. Once at your destination, make your meal and your program your number one priority.

If your breakfast is going to be delayed, do not be tempted to grab "just a little something to tide you over" until you get to your feast, or you will defeat the benefits that a Big Balanced Breakfast can bring. Within a few days of your start on the program, you should find that you have far less trouble waiting for breakfast. Until that time, if you find that holding off presents a bit of a challenge, check out our tips and strategies in Stress-Eating Busters (Chapter 41). You'll find some creative solutions that can make it a snap to hold off until you're ready to feast.

If at all possible, do not reach for a cup of coffee or tea (neither regular nor decaffeinated) until that moment when you're ready to enjoy it with breakfast. Certainly, it is true that these beverages, when taken without sugar or milk, contain no calories. It is *not* the calories that we are concerned with here, however.

Once you've had that cup of coffee or tea, the very pleasure or relief that you experience is a sign that you've already changed your hormonal balance. If you simply *must* have your coffee first thing in the morning, consider having breakfast at home alongside your first cup of coffee or tea. You'll be able to luxuriate, have the coffee boost you crave, fulfill the Big Balanced Breakfast guideline, and get the jump on eliminating your stress-hunger, cravings, and stress-eating for the rest of the day, all at the same time!

If, on the other hand, a homemade breakfast is *not* an option and an early morning cup of coffee or tea is an *absolute* must, down your coffee or tea within the span of a few minutes. Don't linger over it. Then, try to eat your full breakfast as soon as possible.

## Suppose I simply don't have time for breakfast?

No time for breakfast! No desire for breakfast! No worries! The aim of this program is to free you from stress-eating. You can't relieve stress-eating if you continue to endure a stress-producing schedule of responsibilities. If you're not able to have a Big Balanced Breakfast because of your commitment to others, we urge you to consider that your success in this program or any other important endeavor in your life may mean putting your own needs, dreams, and desires first.

If, however, you absolutely *cannot* make time for breakfast, if getting up or out of the house early is not possible because of other uncompromising obligations, you can always choose to enjoy an Alternative Meal in place of a Big Balanced Breakfast. You'll find a full description and samples below.

## Suppose I just don't want breakfast?

We'd love you to *try* having breakfast for a few days. In many cases, your dislike of or disinterest in breakfast is actually a function of either your hormonal imbalance or a pattern of eating that guarantees you'll be indulging yourself by the end of the day.

So if at all possible, give it a chance. If you don't like breakfast foods, include foods you usually eat later in the day (in balance, of course!). Can't eat too early? Hold off and enjoy your breakfast at the first sign of hunger, but still make it the first meal of the day.

If, on the other hand, a Big Balanced Breakfast is a definite no-show, read over the description of the Alternative Meal on the next page, see the samples that follow, and consider the Alternative Meal as fulfillment of this step's guideline.

# What is an Alternative Meal?

We know that not everyone is a breakfast eater. Some folks just find a Big Balanced Breakfast remarkably unappealing. For others, there simply is no time during the workweek for a Big Balanced Breakfast (and/or no desire for it on weekends).

For those who prefer a Big Balanced Breakfast, there may be times, as well, when it is simply not a feasible option or when a luxurious meal at the end of the day would be far more enjoyable. Holidays, celebrations, and vacations can, likewise, rule out a Big Balanced Breakfast.

If you would like to pass on a Big Balanced Breakfast in general or only on occasion, you are welcome on any day (or all days) to choose an Alternative Meal in its place.

The Alternative Meal is a daily, balanced meal that takes the place of the Big Balanced Breakfast. It may be eaten at any time later in the day or evening.

The time that an Alternative Meal is eaten can vary from day to day, as you desire. Enjoy a wonderful dinner out on Saturday night, complete with wine and chocolate soufflé. On Sunday, share in the celebration of a wedding luncheon. On Monday, return to your Big Balanced Breakfast or, if you prefer, an Alternative Meal at dinnertime once again.

Both the Big Balanced Breakfast and the Alternative Meal should contain equal portions of Balancing Foods and Comfort Foods.

*Important Note:* If you choose an Alternative Meal instead of a Big Balanced Breakfast, continue eating your usual breakfast (or not eating breakfast) as you had been doing prior to starting the program.

Be certain to apply all future guidelines to your usual, *non*–Big Balanced Breakfast.

The Alternative Meal differs from the Big Balanced Breakfast in one important aspect: Later, in Step #3, you will be asked to add Balancing Vegetables and Salad to your Alternative Meals (but *not* to Big Balanced Breakfasts).

When you enjoy an Alternative Meal in place of a Big Balanced Breakfast, continue eating the breakfast you used to have before you began the program. If you used to have a bagel, have it. If you used to have cold cereal, enjoy. For the purposes of future steps, each of these choices is considered a *non*–Big Balanced Breakfast.

While choosing Alternative Meals, if you're used to having just a cup of coffee or skipping breakfast, continue. For purposes of future steps, these choices should *not* be considered a *non*–Big Balanced Breakfast. No changes need to be made to them.

## JUST IN CASE

If you include an Alternative Meal as a regular part of your regular program, it is quite possible that you may reap the same benefits as you would from a Big Balanced Breakfast. If you do, that's terrific!

If, on the other hand, when you have completed all seven steps of the program, you find that you are *not* experiencing a remarkable freedom from stress-hunger, cravings, and stress-eating, or if your weight loss slows or reaches a plateau, we urge you to consider making time for a Big Balanced Breakfast as a regular part of your program.

## FINE-TUNING STEP #1

With the addition of a Big Balanced Breakfast or Alternative Meal at this step, you may feel less stress-hunger and fewer cravings. At any meal or snack *other* than your Big Balanced Breakfast or Alternative Meal, feel free to decrease portion sizes of Comfort Foods. You can skip snacks at any time.

# STEP #1: SAMPLE MEAL PLANS[1]

**Guideline:** Begin each day with a Big Balanced Breakfast (or, if desired, enjoy an Alternative Meal later in the day or evening).

## SAMPLE BIG BALANCED BREAKFAST #1

Cheese omelet[2]
Toast with butter, margarine, and/or jam
Breakfast ham, Canadian bacon, or sausage[3]
Plain yogurt with fresh strawberries
Cheese Danish
Sparkling water, tea, or coffee[4]

## SAMPLE BIG BALANCED BREAKFAST #2

Bagel, lox, and cream cheese[3]
2 scrambled eggs[2]
Cold or hot cereal with milk
Cinnamon scone or doughnut
Sparkling water, tea, or coffee[4]

## SAMPLE ALTERNATIVE MEAL: LUNCH

(in place of a Big Balanced Breakfast)

Chicken sandwich on a submarine roll
with lettuce, tomato, and pickle
2 devilled eggs[5]
Potato chips[6]
Coleslaw
Chocolate cake
Sparkling water, tea, or coffee[4]

---

[1] Sample Meal Plans are intended to illustrate the impact of guidelines on meal choices. They should not be used in place of an eating plan of your own design that is in keeping with the guidelines.

[2] Or the equivalent in egg whites (low-fat or regular cheese, as appropriate)

[3] Low-fat or regular, as appropriate

[4] Feel free to add sugar and cream to your beverage as you like.

[5] Or equivalent in low-fat meat, poultry, milk, or other Balancing Protein.

[6] Baked, low-fat, or regular, as appropriate

# SAMPLE ALTERNATIVE MEAL: LUNCH/DINNER
### (in place of a Big Balanced Breakfast)

**Pizza**
Meatballs or rotisserie chicken
Celery and carrot sticks with onion dip
Mixed nuts
Brownie
Sparkling water, tea, or coffee[4]

# SAMPLE ALTERNATIVE MEAL: DINNER
### (in place of a Big Balanced Breakfast)

Jumbo shrimp cocktail or antipasto
Tossed salad with blue cheese dressing
Turf and Surf (Steak with sautéed mushrooms,
lobster tail with melted butter and garlic)

or

Chicken with mushroom gravy
Green beans amandine
Pie à la mode
Champagne, wine, or beer
Sparkling water, tea, or coffee[4]

With 2 days of Big Balanced Breakfasts (or Alternative Meals) under your belt, you're ready to move on to Step #2!

# 25

# Step #2:
# Building Balance

## GUIDELINE:

### Include Balancing Protein
### in every meal and snack.

While adding this guideline, continue to enjoy a Big Balanced Breakfast or Alternative Meal each day (as per guideline from Step #1).

The changes you will make in this step build on the addition of your Big Balanced Breakfast (or Alternative Meal). Together, Steps #1 and #2 help balance your hormone levels and put your stress-hunger, cravings, and stress-eating on hold.

While you continue to follow the guideline from Step #1 and enjoy a Big Balanced Breakfast (or Alternative Meal) every day, you can easily incorporate this second step into your program.

Balancing Proteins, especially those that are low in saturated fat, can help stabilize your hormone levels and keep them steady throughout the day. As you know, hormonal imbalances set off stress-hunger and cravings that lead to stress-eating. To offset some of the hormonal swings that can set off stress-eating, it's important to include the power of Balancing Proteins.

1. In this step, you will be making choices from the list of Balancing Proteins on pages 244–46.

2. As a starting point, in every meal, include enough Balancing Protein to ensure that each meal contains an *average-size* portion of protein (more about *average-size* in a moment). Later, you will be guided in adjusting quantities (see "Frequently Offered Answers for Frequently Asked Questions" and "Fine-Tuning" in this chapter).

3. As a starting point, in every snack, include enough Balancing Protein to ensure that each snack contains about *half* of an average-size portion of protein. Later, you will be guided in adjusting quantities (see "Frequently Offered Answers for Frequently Asked Questions" and "Fine-Tuning" in this chapter).

4. Give yourself a day to get adjusted to this new addition and a day to iron out the wrinkles.

   If, in 2 days, you have been able to include Balancing Protein in every meal and snack without any difficulties, you're ready to move on to the next step. If you run into challenges, however, or if you find it difficult to fit the addition of Balancing Proteins into your schedule, if you can't seem to find any Balancing Proteins that are appealing, or if you miss even one meal or snack, continue for a short time at this step until you get it right for 2 full days.

*Take the time you need to get it right,*
*but don't linger too long. There's more to come.*

5. If you haven't done so already, read through Chapter 41, Stress-Eating Busters. The information on Comfort Food Act-Alikes can help ensure your ease and success with the program and your weight loss.

   In this step, you will continue to eat as you have been eating in Step #1. You will have both a Big Balanced Breakfast (or Alternative Meal) and your usual meals or snacks. At your Big Balanced Breakfast (or Alternative Meal), you've already been including a healthy portion of Balancing Protein (Step #1). Now, in this step, you'll make certain that you are also including some Balancing Protein in all of your other meals and snacks.

## CHOOSE WISELY

For all of your meals and snacks, whenever possible, choose Balancing Proteins that are low in saturated fat. The higher the saturated fat content of a Balancing Protein, the more likely it is to set off a hormonal imbalance that can lead to stress-eating or slow your weight loss. And that's in addition to the many health concerns connected to dietary saturated fats.

You'll find a quick guide to saturated fats on page 253. To get to your goal faster and make it far easier along the way, and for the sake of your health as well, make sure to refer to the guide and choose Balancing Proteins that are low in saturated fat whenever you can.

## FREQUENTLY OFFERED ANSWERS FOR FREQUENTLY ASKED QUESTIONS

In a moment, we'll give you some simple guidelines for determining how much Balancing Protein you should include in your meals and snacks.

For now, keep in mind that including a huge portion is neither necessary nor desirable. It is important, however, to be consistent; include *some* Balancing Protein in every meal and snack.

If a meal or snack contains quite a bit of Balancing Protein already, you do *not* need to add more.

If a meal contains only a small portion of protein, increase the size of the portion to make it at least an average-size portion.

We know that there is a wide range in what one person thinks of as an average-size portion and what another person considers to be average.

As a rule of thumb, imagine that you are going out to eat at a mid-range restaurant—a local neighborhood diner, perhaps. Imagine what you would expect to get as a serving of meat, chicken, or fish on your lunch or dinner plate. Using that portion size as a starting point, make certain that *all* of your meals (including your Big Balanced Breakfast) contain *at least* an average-size portion of Balancing Protein.

Your snacks should contain about half an average-size portion of Balancing Protein.

Feel like including two different kinds of Balancing Proteins in the same meal? That's terrific. It's a great way to keep your meals varied and interesting. The size of the combined portions should be equal to that which you'd have if you were eating a single Balancing Protein.

If you are eating snacks or meals that contain an average-size portion of Balancing Proteins already, there is no need to add more.

*If you feel that you're eating too much food,*
*cut back equally on both Comfort Foods*
*and Balancing Proteins.*

Before we look at this step in action, let's consider the possibility of too much of a good thing. While *some* Balancing Protein is a good thing, too much is *not* better.

In general, keep the total amount of Balancing Protein at a meal within the average-size range and snacks to about half that size (unless otherwise appropriate for health considerations).

## REAL LIFE, REAL EASY

Here's how this guideline plays out. Suppose that you would normally have some fruit for a snack in the middle of the afternoon. It gives you a pick-me-up, and it's something you look forward to. You usually don't have anything else to eat with it.

To fulfill the guideline for Step #2, you could add about half of an average-size portion of Cheddar cheese (regular or low-fat) to this snack. (It's no coincidence that Europeans serve cheese with their fruit. It helps balance the fruit sugar.)

You may choose to add the same types of Balancing Protein each day or make a different selection depending on your mood and preference.

The sample meal plans that follow will provide you with some practical ways of including Balancing Protein in a typical daily menu. Please don't follow this menu *per se*. It is meant to illustrate how *one day's* menu can change as you add Balancing Proteins.

# STEP #2: SAMPLE MEAL PLANS[1]

**Guideline:** Include Balancing Protein in every meal and snack.

## BIG BALANCED BREAKFAST

(This meal requires no change in order to comply with this guideline.)

Cheese omelet[2]

Toast with butter, margarine, and/or jam

Breakfast ham, Canadian bacon, or sausage[3]

Plain yogurt with fresh strawberries

Danish

Sparkling water, tea, or coffee[4]

## OLD LUNCH

(Prior to starting program)

Chicken noodle soup with roll and butter/margarine

Soda (regular)[5]

Large chocolate chip cookie

## NEW LUNCH

Chicken noodle soup with roll and butter/margarine

Soda (regular)[5]

Large chocolate chip cookie

**ADD**

$1/4$ rotisserie chicken

## OLD MIDAFTERNOON SNACK

(Prior to starting program)

1 to 2 pieces fresh fruit

---

[1] Sample Meal Plans are intended to illustrate the impact of guidelines on meal choices. They should not be used in place of an eating plan of your own design that is in keeping with the guidelines.
[2] Or the equivalent in egg whites (low-fat or regular cheese, as appropriate)
[3] Low-fat or regular, as appropriate
[4] Feel free to add sugar and cream to your beverage, as you like.

## New Midafternoon Snack
1 to 2 pieces fresh fruit
### ADD
Wedge of Cheddar cheese ball coated with nuts[3]

## Old Dinner
(Prior to starting program)
Spaghetti with sauce and garlic bread
Glass of wine
Fresh fruit

## New Dinner
Spaghetti with sauce and garlic bread
Glass of wine
Fresh fruit
### ADD
1 or 2 meatballs

## Old Evening Snack
(Prior to starting program)

Potato chips[6]
Chocolate bar

## New Evening Snack

Potato chips[6]
Chocolate bar
### ADD
3 or 4 Buffalo chicken drumettes

---

[5] Soda and other beverages that are sweetened with sugar or any type of sugar substitute should be considered Comfort Foods and balanced with Balancing Foods. See pages 139 and 225–28.
[6] Baked, low-fat, or regular, as appropriate

# FINE-TUNING

With the inclusion of Balancing Proteins at meals and snacks, you may feel less stress-hunger and fewer cravings. Remember, you are free to decrease portion sizes of Balancing Proteins at any time but be sure to decrease an equal amount of Comfort Foods as well. You can skip snacks at any time.

As you begin to include Balancing Protein in all of your meals and snacks, you may find that you're eating more food than you're used to. Remember that the quantity of the Balancing Protein you add is up to you. Ideally, you will consume an "average" portion at your meals and a half portion at snacks. You can add less protein, though, if that's your preference or if limiting protein is necessary to stay within your health requirements.

If you are enjoying the protein and *naturally* want to reduce the Comfort Foods you eat at that meal or snack—not because you *have* to, but because you *want* to—feel free to go a little lighter on your Comfort Food portions.

In the same way, if you are quite hungry at a particular meal or snack, you can choose larger portions of all foods at that meal or snack. Don't just increase the portion size of your Comfort Foods, however; increase all of the foods equally.

As you can see, the size of portions is less important than you might expect. Consistency is essential. As long as you're not compromising your health with inappropriate, unwise, or extreme choices, you can vary portion size.

*Plan the flight, fly the plan.*

Before you begin this step, plan your choices for the next few days. Run through the meals and snacks you might expect to eat and consider which Balancing Proteins you would like to include. Make certain that you have those Balancing Proteins on hand and prepared in a variety of ways to bring you pleasure.

Taking control of your eating can empower you to change your life. Delicious foods bring you pleasure. It's no coincidence that these two feelings, power and pleasure, are two of the best stress-fighters in the world!

# 26

# Step #3:
# Boosting Balance

## GUIDELINE:

**Include Balancing Vegetables
and/or Salad in every lunch, dinner,
Alternative Meal, and snack (but only if
you desire in any breakfast[1]).**

While adding this guideline, continue to enjoy a Big Balanced Breakfast or Alternative Meal each day and include Balancing Proteins in all meals and snacks (as per guidelines from Steps #1 and #2).

Even without the power of protein, the fiber found in vegetables can help stabilize your hormone levels. When fiber gets a chance to combine with protein's hormone-balancing effects, however, the results are excellent!

When Balancing Proteins and Balancing Vegetables and Salad are combined in the right proportions, they can help to stabilize hormone levels throughout the day and night. Together, this dynamic combo can buffer you against the onset of stress-hunger, cravings, and stress-eating and can help keep you in a fat-burning (rather than a fat-making) mode.

If you want to multiply the benefits of the Balancing Proteins that you have added to your meals and snacks, Balancing Vegetables and Salad are a sure bet.

---

[1] There is no need to include Balanced Vegetables and/or Salad at your Big Balanced Breakfast or in your non–Big Balanced Breakfast unless you desire.

To fulfill this step's guideline:

1. Continue enjoying your Big Balanced Breakfast (or Alternative Meal) every day (Step #1). Keep including the Balancing Proteins you added to your lunch, dinner, and snacks (Step #2).

2. For this step, use the Balancing Vegetables and Salad List on page 247 as a guide. Include at least an average serving of vegetables and/or salad with all meals and snacks *other than* your Big Balanced Breakfast.

   On any day that you eat an Alternative Meal, include Balancing Vegetables and Salad in your Alternative Meal, but it is *not* necessary to include them in your usual breakfast (unless you desire).

3. Use the local diner rule from Step #2 for estimating an average serving of vegetables. That is, consider the portion size you would expect to be served at your local diner as an average-size portion. Make certain that an average-size serving of Balancing Vegetables and Salad is included in each meal and at least half that size in every snack.

   Certainly, within reason, feel free to add more than an average serving of Balancing Vegetables and Salad. Remember, only those vegetables that are included on the list on page 247 should be considered Balancing Foods.

   Though it is not necessary, it's a great idea to add some Balancing Vegetables or Salad to your Big Balanced Breakfast as well. Cool cucumber is often a refreshing breakfast side. We love it with a bit of plain yogurt.

   If you feel like adding a variety of Balancing Vegetables or salad makings to a meal, that's wonderful!

   If you are eating snacks or meals that already contain an average-size portion of Balancing Vegetables and Salad, there is no need to add more (though you may).

   It's important to keep in mind that, while you are making certain that Balancing Vegetables and Salad are included in your meals and snacks, you are free to enjoy all of the Comfort Foods you would normally include in these meals as well.

4. Take a day to work out the kinks on these new additions. Take another to make certain you can do it with ease.

In 2 days, if you have been able to include Balancing Vegetables and Salad without any difficulties, you're ready to move on to the next step. If you've missed even one meal or snack (other than your Big Balanced Breakfast, at which it's an option), or if you can't seem to find any Balancing Vegetables or Salad that are appealing, continue for a short time at this step until you get it right for 2 days.

*Overcooked, unadorned, tasteless vegetables
can turn a veggie-lover into a veggie-hater.*

## NEVER EAT A NAKED VEGETABLE

Make certain the Balancing Vegetables and/or Salad you include in your meals are really tasty and satisfying. It does you no good to attempt to force down a mountain of mushy vegetables or tasteless fiber. You may be motivated, but you can put up with that sort of unpleasantness for only so long.

Instead, we urge you to be creative. Think of all the ways you can make vegetables appealing and fun. Stir-fry some green beans with pine nuts; top asparagus with a smooth cheese sauce (regular or low-fat); surround a sour cream dip with broccoli florets, celery sticks, and mushrooms; or stuff some mushrooms with crushed almonds browned in olive oil.

Spice up your salads with shredded cheese, browned beef, and spices, and you instantly have a delicious taco salad. Add some julienned meats and cheese to a salad, toss with blue cheese dressing, and you have a satisfying Cobb salad that is yours for the taking.

A stir-fried shrimp or a chicken, tuna, beef, or pork salad added to your lunch can take the ho-hum out of the meal. Celery stuffed with cream cheese can make a great grab-and-go snack all by itself. You'll find some fun tips, ideas, and recipes in Chapter 43. For starters, though, we'll tell you what has worked for us for more than 25 years.

*We never met a vegetable we didn't like.*
*We ran too fast for them to catch up.*

We started out as veggie-haters or, more accurately, veggie-avoiders. When Rachael weighed more than 300 pounds (for more than 30 years of her life), her idea of a salad was a tiny, wilted piece of lettuce placed squarely in the center of a 3-inch-thick sandwich.

As a very chubby kid, Richard grew up thinking that if you included some corn, baked beans, or potatoes in your dinner, you had more than met your nutritional need for vegetables.

Together, we discovered the Secret to Vegetable Taming: That is, *never, ever eat a naked vegetable.*

Dip it, wrap it, stir-fry it, cover it, or tuck it in between layers of protein. Add sauces or salad dressings, meats, cheeses, sour cream or yogurt (be sure that your choices are low in saturated fat); spice it up, dip it in crushed nuts, and sauté it in olive oil—do whatever you must or whatever you like within the context of this program and good common sense, but, whatever you do, don't ever force yourself to eat a naked vegetable.

Unless you love vegetables to begin with, eating plain, steamed vegetables is enough to make you avoid them for a long time. If pure veggie eating brings you pleasure, so much the better. You're a very fortunate person.

If, on the other hand, veggie loving is not an inborn instinct, take on the Veggie Challenge and make them taste good—really good—for the sake of your hormonal balance, your weight, your health, and your longevity.

# You Don't Have to Eat the Whole Cauliflower

The quantity of vegetables or salad that you add to each meal or snack is not as important as being consistent with your vegetable intake.

If you can, and you are willing to do so, the addition of one full average serving of vegetables and/or salad to every lunch and dinner, and at least half that amount in each snack, is ideal. Adding two different vegetables or both a vegetable and a salad to a meal is a great way to be sure you're getting a good supply of fiber, although anything more than an average serving is strictly a matter of choice.

Don't strive for perfection, and don't push yourself to the point where you feel like rebelling. The challenge is not to force yourself to eat the vegetables but to make them so good that you *want* to eat them.

## FINE-TUNING STEP #3

With the inclusion of Balancing Vegetables and/or Salad at meals and snacks, you may feel less stress-hunger and fewer cravings. At any meal or snack *other* than your Big Balanced Breakfast or Alternative Meal, feel free to decrease portion sizes of Comfort Foods. You can skip snacks at any time.

While you're fine-tuning this step, consider fine-tuning your program in general. Now might be a good time to add a Hormone-Balancing Activity or Adventure to your day. Read Chapter 41, Stress-Eating Busters, for some unique and fun suggestions.

## CHOICE EXAMPLES

We'll take a look at the way in which the guideline for Step #3 plays out in real life, but first, a clarification: For purposes of illustration, our examples incorporate the same foods every day.

In this way, we can best show how a meal changes with each successive step. The meals we describe or include in our examples are used as illustrations only, and because of that, they don't vary from day to day.

You, on the other hand, should choose from a wide variety of Balancing Vegetables and Salads and Balancing Proteins.

Here are some examples of the changes you might make as you incorporate Step #3 into your daily eating program.

# STEP #3: SAMPLE MEAL PLANS[2]

**Guideline:** Include Balancing Vegetables and Salad
in every meal and snack (but only if you desire in any breakfast).

## BIG BALANCED BREAKFAST

(This meal requires no change in order to comply with this guideline.)

Cheese omelet[3]
Toast with butter, margarine, and/or jam
Breakfast ham, Canadian bacon, or sausage[4]
Plain yogurt with fresh strawberries
Danish
Sparkling water, tea, or coffee[5]

## OLD LUNCH

(Using prior guidelines)

Chicken noodle soup with roll and butter/margarine
$1/4$ rotisserie chicken
Soda (regular)[6]
Large chocolate chip cookie

## NEW LUNCH

Chicken noodle soup with roll and butter/margarine
$1/4$ rotisserie chicken
Soda (regular)[6]
Large chocolate chip cookie
Side salad (lettuce, mushrooms, green peppers,
and cucumber) with buttermilk dressing

## OLD MIDAFTERNOON SNACK

(Using prior guidelines)

1 or 2 pieces fresh fruit
Wedge of Cheddar cheese and nut ball[4]

---

[2] Sample Meal Plans are intended to illustrate the impact of the guidelines on meal choices. They should not be used in place of an eating plan of your own design that is in keeping with the guidelines.

[3] Or the equivalent in egg whites (low-fat or regular cheese, as appropriate)

[4] Low-fat or regular, as appropriate

## New Midafternoon Snack

1 or 2 pieces fresh fruit
Wedge of Cheddar cheese and nut ball[4]
Sour cream garlic dip with finger salad vegetables[7]

## Old Dinner

(Using prior guidelines)

Spaghetti with sauce, 1 or 2 meatballs, and garlic bread
Glass of wine
Fresh fruit

## New Dinner

Spaghetti with sauce, 1 or 2 meatballs, and garlic bread
Glass of wine
Fresh fruit
Asparagus spears amandine

## Old Evening Snack

(Using prior guidelines)

Potato chips
Chocolate bar
3 or 4 Buffalo chicken drumettes

## New Evening Snack

Potato chips
Chocolate bar
3 or 4 Buffalo chicken drumettes
Cucumber slices, celery sticks, mushroom caps,
and green pepper slices with blue cheese dip[4]

---

[5] Feel free to add sugar and cream to your beverage, as you like.

[6] Soda and other beverages that are sweetened with sugar or any type of sugar substitute should be considered Comfort Foods and balanced with Balancing Foods. See pages 139 and 225–28.

[7] Celery sticks, green pepper, cucumbers, or any selection from the Balancing Vegetables and Salad List on page 247.

# FROM TOO MUCH TO JUST RIGHT

As you begin adding vegetables and salad to your lunch, dinner, and snacks, you may be keenly aware of eating more food than you're used to. What had been a snack may begin to look like a small meal.

It may taste very good, and you may choose to eat it all. That's up to you. As long as the meal or snack is balanced, it is yours to enjoy.

> *You may suddenly discover*
> *you don't want that much food!*
> *How delightful!*

Within a short time on this program, however, you may discover that you simply don't *want* to eat that much food; if you think it unwise or unpleasant, then don't! There is always another meal just around the bend.

If you do reduce the quantity of your food, however, be very certain to reduce all of the food equally. In other words, if you reduce the portion of Balancing Protein or Balancing Vegetables and Salad that you've included, reduce the portion of Comfort Food that you're eating as well.

You may be surprised at how quickly your cravings for Comfort Foods drop as the power of the fiber in Balancing Vegetables and Salad combines with Balancing Protein to keep your hormones in check.

If you are enjoying your Balancing Protein, Vegetables, and Salad and *naturally* want to reduce your Comfort Food intake for that meal or snack, feel free to take a bit less Comfort Food right then, or if you choose, leave a little Comfort Food behind. Snacks are a matter of choice. If you don't need them anymore, you can skip them. Listen to your body as it returns to balance.

# 27

# Step #4:
# Winning at Losing

## GUIDELINE:

### At all snacks, eat Balancing Foods only.

While adding this guideline, continue to enjoy a Big Balanced Breakfast or Alternative Meal each day and include Balancing Proteins and Vegetables and Salad[1] in all meals and snacks (as per guidelines from Steps #1 to #3).

This guideline can help bring your body into the final stage of balance. It is designed to help you enter a fat-burning, weight-loss mode and remain there longer.

When you eat Comfort Foods frequently, throughout the day, your body experiences these foods as stresses in themselves. The hormone imbalance that results pulls you into a Stress-Eating Pattern, which signals your body to shift into a fat-making and fat-storing mode. This is your body's Saving Mode, when your metabolism slows down to keep you from burning energy while your Stress-Eating Pattern prompts you to keep bringing in more food.

The more often you eat Comfort Food, the more often your body shifts into your Stress-Eating Pattern and Saving Mode, the longer you remain there, the more difficult it is to lose weight and the easier it is to gain it.

If you ever thought that all you had to do to gain weight was just look at food, you may not have been far from the truth.

---

[1] There is no need to include Balanced Vegetables and/or Salad at your Big Balanced Breakfast or in your non–Big Balanced Breakfast unless you desire.

Depending on your particular pattern of stress-eating, just the thought, sight, and, certainly, the smell of your favorite Comfort Food can set off a cascade of hormones that will begin to make fat from the blood sugar you have in your body—even though you might not ever take a single bite of the Comfort Food!

*The reigning wisdom states that 3,500 calories*
*equals a pound of fat (lost or gained).*
*Not necessarily! Not for everyone!*

Once you are trapped in a Saving Mode, it can be an uphill battle to start the weight-loss ball rolling. In this no-man's-land, the old 3,500-calories-equals-a-pound rule simply does not hold.

You can eat only 1,000 calories above what your body needs and put on several pounds (not just water weight). You can eat 6,000 or 7,000 calories less than what your body needs and not lose a pound. To lose weight at a predictable and rewarding pace, you have to get your body out of its Saving Mode and into a Spending Mode.

To keep losing weight at a steady rate, you need to stay in the Spending Mode as long as possible while getting the nutrition you need to stay healthy. At the same time, you must be sure to get the pleasure you need to stay motivated.

Fortunately, you can do both without difficulty.

In the previous step, you learned to balance your Comfort Foods, Balancing Proteins, and Balancing Vegetables and Salads. That guideline readied your body to begin to decrease the frequency with which you take in Comfort Foods.

Now, Step #4's guideline will help you use the Frequency Factor to avoid falling into your particular Stress-Eating Pattern and, at the same time, to move into your Spending Mode and lose weight.

In this step, you will reduce the number of times each day you eat Comfort Food and, in doing so, reduce the *frequency* with which your body experiences the hormonal messages that catapult it into a Savings Mode.

*Seventy-five percent of calories are burned while you're at rest.*
*The goal is to keep spending energy though you're not doing a thing!*

The longer the times between eating Comfort Food, the longer your body stays in a Spending Mode. The longer your body stays in a Spending Mode, the greater your weight loss, the less hunger you feel, and the fewer cravings. You will still be able to eat the Comfort Foods you love in the quantities you desire. You're just going to hold off and save them for your meals.

So, if you've ever said, "I could stay on a diet, really stick with it, if I could just have the food I love *sometimes*," here's your chance.

For Step #4, you are asked to save all of your Comfort Foods for meals only. In other words, no Comfort Foods during snacks.

If you are uncertain as to what constitutes a meal versus a snack, use the following as a guide: Your three largest intakes of food per day are meals. Anything else is a snack, and during these snacks, don't have any Comfort Foods.

As you follow this guideline while continuing to follow all prior guidelines, you should have Comfort Foods three times a day only. As you enjoy Balancing Proteins and Balancing Vegetables and Salad at your snacks, you'll be spending more time burning fat instead of socking it away in your fat cells.

Not a bad deal at all.

## COMFORT FOODS APLENTY

A guideline that asks you to save your Comfort Foods for another time is *not* asking you to give up a full and satisfying snack or meal. When you remove your Comfort Foods from a snack or, in the future, in a meal, you are welcome to replace those Comfort Foods with additional Balancing Proteins and Balancing Vegetables and Salad. Just keep the additions within the limits of previous guidelines.

## BEVERAGES

In this step, you begin to save your Comfort Foods and enjoy them at any meal (but not at snacks). As you progress to the next guideline, you will be asked to save your Comfort Foods and enjoy them at *some* of your meals only (and not at any snacks). Meals and snacks that do not contain Comfort Foods will be made up of Balancing Proteins and Balancing Vegetables and Salad only.

When it comes to beverages, consider the following: During the meals and snacks that contain no Comfort Foods and in between, as well, it would be very helpful to avoid beverages that contain either sugar or sugar substitutes. When it comes to hormone balance, stress-hunger, cravings, stress-eating, and weight concerns, sugar substitutes can create more problems than the sugar they are meant to replace.

You'll find some remarkable new information on sugar substitutes, along with a proven method for kicking the sugar substitute habit, on page 225. We urge you to read this brief section and consider what it has to say. Wouldn't it be a shame to allow so-called diet drinks to keep you stuck in a Stress-Eating Cycle and prevent you from losing weight?

# AHEAD OF THE GAME

What should you do if, before you came to this step, you were eating Comfort Foods only three times a day (or less often)? Suppose you were already eating nothing but three meals a day (or fewer)?

In either case, this guideline would require no change on your part.

First, however, it's important to be certain that you are not, in fact, eating Comfort Foods more often than three times a day without realizing that you are doing so. Read over the Comfort Foods List on pages 248–51 very carefully. Read the section on Comfort Food Act-Alikes on pages 225–35 as well. You might be surprised to find that every time you pop some chewing gum or a mint (regular or sugar-free) into your mouth, you are "eating" a Comfort Food. The same goes with fruit juice, power drinks, and sodas, all of which contain either natural sugar, added sugar, or sugar substitute.

Once you have carefully reviewed the Comfort Foods List and the special section on Comfort Food Act-Alikes and you are sure that you have *not* been eating Comfort Foods more than three times a day, you can choose to go to Step #5 immediately and begin to incorporate that guideline into your eating program, if you like.

On the other hand, if you prefer, you can consider that you've just been awarded a mini-vacation from change. You can coast on your hard work and smart choices and, for the next 2 days, just continue with your guidelines as you have been doing.

We strongly suggest that you refrain from putting pressure on yourself in either direction. Just do what you feel like doing. This is your program, your weight loss, your life, and your success.

Many people remember this guideline because within a short amount of time after incorporating it into their eating program, they see the cumulative impact the program has on their stress-hunger, cravings, stress-eating, and weight.

In some cases, however, you might encounter a bit of resistance you did not expect—from yourself! If you have difficulty giving up high-carb foods at all snacks, please be certain you have been following all of the previous guidelines.

The previous guidelines were designed to begin to balance your body in preparation for decreasing the number of times each day you eat Comfort Foods. If you have been fudging on any of the previous guidelines (no pun intended), your body may still be in a state of hormonal imbalance; the greater the hormonal imbalance that remains, the harder it is to eat Comfort Foods less frequently.

If giving up Comfort Foods at your snacks presents a challenge, here's a solution that just might do the trick:

First, reread each of the previous guidelines in order. Slowly. Don't skim. If you need to clean any of them up, stop and take a day or two (or three) to get each guideline right.

On the other hand, if you have been following them as they are written, make sure that you've been giving yourself enough time to take care of getting the food you need when you need it. Taking the time to get yourself the food that will please you and, at the same time, meet the guidelines of each step is essential to your success. Do not just "make do" with whatever Balancing Food you find handy. You deserve more care and attention than that!

Step #4 is an important guideline. It marks a transition into a new level of hormonal balance. Take 2 days to get it right, or a little more time, if needed. Get it right for 2 full days before moving to the next step.

# STEP #4: SAMPLE MEAL PLANS[2]

**Guideline:** At all snacks, eat Balancing Foods only.

## BIG BALANCED BREAKFAST
(This meal requires no change in order to comply with this guideline.)

Cheese omelet[3]
Toast with butter, margarine, and/or jam
Breakfast ham, Canadian bacon, or sausage[4]
Plain yogurt with fresh strawberries
Danish
Sparkling water, tea, or coffee[5]

## LUNCH
(This meal requires no change in order to comply with this guideline.)

Side salad (lettuce, mushrooms, green peppers,
and cucumber) with buttermilk dressing
Chicken noodle soup with roll and butter/margarine
1/4 rotisserie chicken
Soda (regular)[6]
Large chocolate chip cookie

## OLD MIDAFTERNOON SNACK
(Using prior guidelines)

1 piece fresh fruit
Large wedge of Cheddar cheese ball coated with nuts[4]
Sour cream garlic dip with finger salad vegetables[7]

## NEW MIDAFTERNOON SNACK
(*Note:* To comply with this guideline, Comfort Foods were removed
and Balancing Protein added as replacement.)

---

[2] Sample Meal Plans are intended to illustrate the impact of the guidelines on meal choices. They should not be used in place of an eating plan of your own design that is in keeping with the guidelines.
[3] Or the equivalent in egg whites (low-fat or regular cheese, as appropriate)
[4] Low-fat or regular, as appropriate
[5] Feel free to add sugar and cream to your beverage, as you like.

Wedge of Cheddar cheese ball coated with nuts[4]
Sour cream garlic dip with large selection
of finger salad vegetables[7]
Three handfuls of almonds[8]

## DINNER

(This meal requires no change in order to comply with this guideline.)

Garlic bread
Glass of wine
Spaghetti with sauce and 1 or 2 meatballs
Asparagus spears amandine
Fresh fruit

## OLD EVENING SNACK

(Using prior guidelines)

Cucumber slices, celery sticks, mushroom caps,
and green pepper slices with blue cheese dip[4]
Potato chips
Chocolate bar
3 or 4 Buffalo chicken drumettes

## NEW EVENING SNACK

(*Note:* To comply with this guideline, Comfort Foods were removed.
Balancing Foods were added to compensate.)

Cucumber slices, celery sticks, mushroom caps,
and green pepper slices with blue cheese dip[4]
3 or 4 Buffalo chicken drumettes
Wedge of Crustless Mushroom Quiche[9]

---

[6] Soda and other beverages that are sweetened with sugar or any type of sugar substitute should be considered Comfort Foods and balanced with Balancing Foods. See pages 139 and 225–28.

[7] Celery sticks, green pepper, cucumbers, or any selection from the Balancing Vegetables and Salad List on page 247.

[8] Balancing Protein (almonds) added to better approximate equal portions of all three food groups.

[9] See page 256 for recipe.

# 28

# Step #5:
# Heading Into
# the Final Stretch

## GUIDELINE:

### Eat only Balancing Foods
### at all snacks and one meal.

While adding this guideline, continue to enjoy a Big Balanced Breakfast or Alternative Meal each day and include Balancing Proteins and Vegetables and/or Salad[1] in all meals and snacks (as per guidelines from Steps #1, #2, and #3).

Congratulations! You're almost to the last step in your program. With each of the two steps that remain, the benefits, in terms of stress-hunger, cravings, stress-eating, and weight reduction, multiply greatly.

In this step, you will eat only Balancing Foods at all snacks and at one meal. You will save your Comfort Foods for your Big Balanced Breakfast (or Alternative Meal) and for one other meal each day.

Only these two meals each day should contain any Comfort Foods. At all snacks and at any other meals, you will eat only Balancing Proteins and Balancing Vegetables and Salad.

As always, make certain that you take the time and care to please

---

[1] There is no need to include Balancing Vegetables and/or Salad at your Big Balanced Breakfast or in your non–Big Balanced Breakfast unless you desire.

yourself; treat yourself like an honored guest. If it means going an extra few blocks out of your way or spending a few extra dollars, we urge you to splurge on yourself, if at all possible.

Your Big Balanced Breakfast or Alternative Meal will remain the same. For all of your snacks and for any other meals each day, enjoy a healthy balance of Balancing Proteins and Balancing Vegetables or Salad.

It's likely that you've mastered the skills needed for this step as you were practicing the previous guideline. The only difference here is that you will save your Comfort Foods for a total of two meals (including your Big Balanced Breakfast or Alternative Meal) instead of three.

Before your day begins, decide at which meal (in addition to your Big Balanced Breakfast or Alternative Meal) you would like to enjoy your Comfort Foods. Choose any meal you prefer.

*Life is full of unexpected pleasures. You need an eating program that allows you to enjoy them—fully!*

While it is helpful to decide prior to starting your day which meal will contain your Comfort Foods, life is full of surprises; and part of the joy in life is being able to take advantage of the fun that lands, unannounced, at your door.

Imagine, for a moment, that you have decided that, in addition to your Big Balanced Breakfast, you are going to have a quiet but luxurious dinner at home with your mate. The day before, you stock the refrigerator with your favorite foods (both Comfort and Balanced), and all is in readiness.

While at work, you remember that it is a co-worker's birthday; and as the sandwiches and cake appear during your lunch break, you wonder if you can change your choice and enjoy the Comfort Food that is being served at the celebration. The answer is a resounding "yes."

At the celebration, remember to keep the Comfort Food to Balancing Food portions in equal proportion, and simply save the goodies that are waiting at home for tomorrow's Big Balanced Breakfast or Alternative Meal.

*Plan your day, but don't carve it in stone.*

While it is helpful to *plan* for the day, you are, by no means, locked into your decision. Try to avoid spontaneously deciding, in the few moments before you eat, whether or not to include Comfort Foods in that meal. We want you to feel the power of choice that is yours to have or to refrain from having your Comfort Foods depending on what you want and what will bring you the most pleasure.

## BEEN THERE, DOING THAT

If you are already saving your Comfort Foods for two meals a day (or fewer) or if you generally eat nothing other than two meals a day (or fewer), you already meet this guideline.

You can either move to Step #6 (the last step in the program) at this time or you can consider the step to be a short, 2-day stop in which you need to change nothing while continuing to follow all prior guidelines. It's your choice. Choose whichever path pleases you most and is the most stress free!

*Spend, spend, spend.*
*Who knew losing weight could be such fun!*

## SPENDING STRATEGY

The purpose of this guideline and the final guideline that follows in the next chapter is to remain in the Spending Mode to better burn the energy you take in as well as the energy stored in your fat cells. By helping to balance your hormone levels as well, these two guidelines help to decrease your stress-hunger and cravings so that remaining free of a Stress-Eating Cycle becomes easier with each day.

For this step, you are asked to save your Comfort Foods and enjoy them during two meals daily. It's important to remember that when you remove your Comfort Foods from any meal or snack, you are free to replace them with additional Balancing Proteins and Balancing Vegetables and Salad in keeping with previous guidelines.

# TIMING, TIMING, TIMING

This guideline is a direct extension of the previous step. In addition to eating only Balancing Foods at snacks, in this step, you are asked to include only Balancing Foods at one of your meals as well.

You may welcome this change. You may realize that you are that much closer to your weight-loss goal and that as you continue, your stress-hunger, cravings, and stress-eating will continue to disappear.

You may also enjoy a new sense of control and the emerging understanding that what you might formerly have considered to be a lack of willpower was, indeed, a physical imbalance after all.

On the other hand, you may need a little time to adjust to not having Comfort Foods at one of your meals (in addition to not having Comfort Foods at snacks).

*Don't settle for less than ease and pleasure.*
*You have it coming.*

If you had difficulty meeting this step's guideline, give yourself the freedom to experiment with your choice of meals that will include Balancing Foods only; try different types of food as well as different settings in which to eat these meals.

For one person, for example, a Balancing Food lunch might be simple. A big salad with tuna and shredded cheese might be enough to do the trick. For another, however, giving up a full lunch complete with dessert might prove, at this time, too much of a sacrifice.

In the former scenario, lunch was an excellent choice for a Balancing-Foods-only meal to meet today's guideline. In the latter scenario, however, lunch (a special time of stress relief) was not the ideal choice.

So give yourself a little latitude. Take a day or two if you need them to make some good choices. Then you'll be ready to move on to your next (and last) guideline.

# Step #5: Sample Meal Plans[2]

**Guideline:** Eat only Balancing Foods at all snacks and one meal.

## Big Balanced Breakfast
(This meal requires no change in order to comply with this guideline.)

Cheese omelet[3]
Toast with butter, margarine, and/or jam
Breakfast ham, Canadian bacon, or sausage[4]
Plain yogurt with fresh strawberries
Danish
Sparkling water, tea, or coffee[5]

## Old Lunch
(Using prior guidelines)

Side salad (lettuce, mushrooms, green peppers,
and cucumber) with buttermilk dressing
Chicken noodle soup with roll and butter/margarine
$1/4$ rotisserie chicken
Soda (regular)[6]
Large chocolate chip cookie

## New Lunch
(*Note:* To comply with this guideline, Comfort Foods were removed.
Balancing Foods were added or portions increased to compensate.)

Large salad with buttermilk dressing
$1/2$ rotisserie chicken
Baby Bok Choy with Cashews[7]
Seltzer, tea, or coffee[8]

---

[2] Sample Meal Plans are intended to illustrate the impact of the guidelines on meal choices. They should not be used in place of an eating plan of your own design that is in keeping with the guidelines.

[3] Or the equivalent in egg whites (low-fat or regular cheese, as appropriate)

[4] Low-fat or regular, as appropriate

[5] Feel free to add sugar and cream to your beverage, as you like.

[6] Soda and other beverages that are sweetened with sugar or any type of sugar substitute should be considered Comfort Foods and balanced with Balancing Foods. See pages 139 and 225–28.

# MIDAFTERNOON SNACK

(This snack requires no change in order to comply with this guideline.)

Wedge of Cheddar cheese ball coated with nuts[4]
Sour cream garlic dip with large selection
of finger salad vegetables[9]
Three handfuls of almonds

# DINNER

(This meal is the second meal for the day[10] that includes Comfort Foods.
It requires no change in order to comply with this guideline.)

Garlic bread
Glass of wine
Spaghetti with sauce and 1 or 2 meatballs
Asparagus spears amandine
Fresh fruit

# EVENING SNACK

(This snack requires no change in order to comply with this guideline.)

Cucumber slices, celery sticks, mushroom caps,
and green pepper slices with blue cheese dip[4]
3 or 4 Buffalo chicken drumettes
Wedge of Crustless Mushroom Quiche[11]

---

[7] See recipe on page 273.
[8] Feel free to add cream but no sugar to your beverage at this meal.
[9] Celery sticks, green pepper, cucumbers, or any selection from the Balancing Vegetables and Salad List on page 247.
[10] In addition to a Big Balanced Breakfast or Alternative Meal.
[11] See page 256 for recipe.

# 29

# Step #6: Crossing the Finish Line

## GUIDELINE:

### Include Comfort Foods in one meal each day. At all other meals and snacks, eat Balancing Foods only.

While adding this guideline, continue to enjoy a Big Balanced Breakfast or Alternative Meal each day and include Balancing Proteins and Vegetables and/or Salad[1] in all meals and snacks (as per guidelines from Steps #1 to #5).

You've made it! You're here, at the last step in the program! You've overcome all obstacles along the way, and now you are heading into the final stretch. You have only this step to add!

In this step, you will be asked to save your Comfort Foods for your Big Balanced Breakfast or for an Alternative Meal. At all snacks and at all other meals, you will eat only Balancing Proteins and Balancing Vegetables and Salad. You will save your Comfort Foods for one meal each day.

---

[1] There is no need to include Balancing Vegetables and/or Salad at your Big Balanced Breakfast or in your non–Big Balanced Breakfast unless you desire.

With this step come a far greater hormonal balance; a dramatic drop in stress-eating impulses, stress-hunger, and cravings; and a far more predictable weight loss.

When deciding which meal each day will include your Comfort Foods, you may continue to enjoy your Big Balanced Breakfast. As the need arises, you may switch to an Alternative Meal and enjoy your Comfort Foods at lunch or dinner.

We strongly recommend that, as consistently as possible, you continue to confine your once-daily Comfort Food treats to your Big Balanced Breakfast. Try to keep a Big Balanced Breakfast as part of your standard eating program.

When a social event, special evening out, or celebration makes an Alternative Meal a better choice in which to enjoy your Comfort Foods, feel free to switch for that day. As soon as possible, however, try to return to your Big Balanced Breakfast so that you can continue to reap the hormonal benefits it offers.

## PASSING ON A
## BIG BALANCED BREAKFAST

On days that you choose not to have a Big Balanced Breakfast and save your Comfort Foods for an Alternative Meal instead, it is still quite helpful to have a morning meal that consists of Balancing Proteins and Balancing Vegetables and Salad. A mushroom and green pepper omelet might be just perfect, or you could have some nontraditional breakfast foods as well. Got some leftover chicken salad in the refrigerator? Some nice fresh chicken salad can be especially refreshing.

If, on the other hand, nothing appeals to you, perhaps something light such as celery stuffed with cream cheese might do the trick. Whatever you choose for your breakfast on your non–Big Balanced Breakfast day, try to make certain that it's satisfying and filling. Your body is used to a morning feast, and waiting for a later meal may stimulate real (not necessarily stress-related) hunger.

If you find that holding off for a later feast at your Alternative Meal just isn't feasible, it might be better to have that Big Balanced Breakfast after all and change your food choices for the later meal. Be certain, however, that you make special plans to make the later meal extra special (with two different Balancing Proteins, for example) to compensate for the fact that it will not contain any Comfort Foods.

## ONE STEP AHEAD OF THE GAME

If you are already saving your Comfort Foods for one meal a day, you are already meeting this guideline. But there's more to come! In the remaining pages of this chapter, you'll find an important warning along with essential information on personalizing your program to get the maximum results and the maximum pleasure.

## A WARNING TO THE WISE

The eating portion of this program is *not* intended to be a low-carbohydrate eating program. It is intended to change the *frequency* with which you eat carbohydrate-rich and/or high-fat Comfort Foods.

We do not condone, recommend, or suggest refraining from eating carbohydrate-rich foods. Carbohydrate-rich Comfort Foods are needed for good nutrition, for good health, and for satisfaction and balance as well. We strongly recommend that you choose Comfort Foods that are closer to nature, that is, less processed, and that you refrain from consuming foods high in saturated fats or trans fats.

As in all things, your physician's recommendations should outweigh all other considerations.

## ONE LAST STEP

Congratulations! You've made some important changes in a relatively short time. Now, for this last guideline, review the Sample Meal Plans on pages 178 and 179 to help you finish up in style.

## STAYING WITH A WINNER

Once you incorporate this last step of the program, you will be ready to personalize the program to fit your individual needs. Go to the Cure chapter that applies to your particular Stress-Eating Pattern (Chapters 30 through 40). It contains recommendations that will help you get the most out of the program (and with the greatest ease and pleasure).

Within a few days of fulfilling this final guideline and incorporating your personalized recommendations, your need to stress-eat should be eliminated. Should stress-hunger or cravings return, review this step and the food lists on pages 244 through 251 to be certain you are following the program as it has been written.

This final step plus your personalized recommendations summarize the program that you will now follow to remain free of stress-eating and to lose weight at a steady, predictable rate.

## THE FINISH LINE

Now that you are at the finish line, we urge you to keep going and growing in the perfection of your program. The Stress-Eating Busters in Chapter 41 may help you along the way. These tips and strategies can help keep your body in balance and your weight loss steady in the face of future stresses and unexpected challenges.

While, on one hand, you have completed the eating portion of the program, even as you continue to incorporate all of the guidelines that you fulfilled along the way and incorporate your personalized recommendations, you are beginning a whole new adventure.

As your body continues to find balance, your mind and spirit will discover a newfound joy. It's an amazing journey! On many levels, the best is yet to come.

# STEP #6: SAMPLE MEAL PLANS[2]

**Guideline:** Include Comfort Foods in one meal each day.
At all other meals and snacks, eat Balancing Foods only.

## BIG BALANCED BREAKFAST

(This meal requires no change in order to comply with this guideline.)

Cheese omelet[3]
Toast with butter, margarine, and/or jam
Breakfast ham, Canadian bacon, or sausage[4]
Plain yogurt with fresh strawberries
Danish
Sparkling water, tea, or coffee[5]

## LUNCH

(This meal requires no change in order to comply with this guideline.)

Large salad with buttermilk dressing
$1/2$ rotisserie chicken
Baby Bok Choy with Cashews[6]
Seltzer, tea, or coffee[7]

## MIDAFTERNOON SNACK

(This snack requires no change in order to comply with this guideline.)

Wedge of Cheddar cheese ball coated with nuts[4]
Sour cream garlic dip with large selection
of finger salad vegetables[8]
Three handfuls of almonds

---

[2] Sample Meal Plans are intended to illustrate the impact of the guidelines on meal choices. They should not be used in place of an eating plan of your own design that is in keeping with the guidelines.

[3] Or the equivalent in egg whites (low-fat or regular cheese, as appropriate)

[4] Low-fat or regular, as appropriate

[5] Feel free to add sugar and cream to your beverage, as you like.

[6] See recipe on page 273.

[7] Feel free to add cream but no sugar to your beverage at this meal.

# OLD DINNER

Garlic bread

Glass of wine

Spaghetti with sauce and 1 or 2 meatballs

Asparagus spears amandine

Fresh fruit

# NEW DINNER

(*Note:* Comfort Food items were removed to comply with this guideline.
Balancing Foods were added to compensate.)

Jumbo shrimp cocktail or antipasto

Artichoke spinach dip with crudités[8]

3 or 4 meatballs

*or*

Surf and Turf: Steak with sautéed mushrooms,
lobster tail with melted butter and garlic

Asparagus spears amandine

Seltzer, tea, or coffee[7]

# EVENING SNACK

(This snack requires no change in order to comply with this guideline.)

Cucumber slices, celery sticks, mushroom caps,
and green pepper slices with blue cheese dip[4]

3 or 4 Buffalo chicken drumettes

Wedge of Crustless Mushroom Quiche[9]

---

[8] Celery sticks, green pepper, cucumbers, or any selection from the Balancing Vegetables and Salad List on page 247.
[9] See page 256 for recipe.

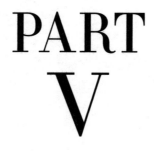

# PART
# V

# 30

# The Frustration-Induced Stress-Eater's Cure

## Your Personalized Plan

### Getting Started

The recommendations you find within this chapter have been individualized specifically for the Frustration-Induced Stress-Eater. Apply these recommendations to the Stress-Eating Cure Program (Chapters 21 through 29). They will turn the Stress-Eating Cure Program into your personalized Stress-Eating Cure.

To help eliminate their stress-hunger and cravings and to lose weight, Frustration-Induced Stress-Eaters need a personalized plan designed to decrease the levels of adrenaline that flood their bodies while, at the same time, boosting their levels of oxytocin.

*As you balance one hormone, the others*
*will fall into balance naturally.*

Fortunately, if you are a Frustration-Induced Stress-Eater, the Stress-Eating Cure Program, preferably the Quick-Start Plan[1] (as described in

---

[1] Either the Quick-Start Plan or the Step-by-Step Plan can bring you the results you desire. The Quick-Start Plan is more challenging and yields more immediate results.

Chapter 22), can help you balance one hormone simply by balancing the other.

Researchers have not been able to discover a reliable way in which to lower adrenaline levels directly without the use of extreme drug-induced states. Instead, the most effective way to reduce adrenaline appears to be by increasing adrenaline's competitive hormone, oxytocin.

This scientific finding works perfectly for the Frustration-Induced Stress-Eater, who, by definition, needs to do both!

If you are a Frustration-Induced Stress-Eater, the best way to raise oxytocin levels is to think "back to basics." Experiences that give you a sense of security, relief, and joy are often those that raise levels of this hormone.

Physical contact—platonic or sexual in nature with someone you feel connected to—massage, self-massage, and masturbation have all been shown to raise oxytocin levels. Simple things, like snuggling in your favorite blanket, getting a satisfying back scratch, brushing your hair with a pleasantly stiff brush, even brushing your teeth, can all help bring your hormone levels back into balance.

*Your pet can help balance your hormones!*

There are many experiences that do not involve physical contact but do "touch" you emotionally that can raise your oxytocin levels as well. A good talk with a friend, your empathy toward a stranger, an act of kindness, sharing a meal, listening to your favorite soul-satisfying music, singing, playing a musical instrument, the enjoyment of beautiful scenery, deeply pleasurable and reminiscent smells—all can do wonders when it comes to raising your oxytocin levels.

Being with a pet that brings you pleasure, even if you're not petting it, has also been shown to raise oxytocin levels. Studies have shown that being with a beloved pet is as emotionally satisfying as talking with a friend or family member. No wonder people with pets tend to live (and love) longer!

Food choices can have a great effect on oxytocin. Fatty foods release far more oxytocin than most other foods. That's one of the reasons that high-fat, smooth, rich, and creamy foods are so satisfying. Please note that we are not saying the best way to balance your hormones is to eat lots of fatty foods; just the opposite, in fact.

Foods that are high in saturated fats and trans fats are clearly unhealthy choices. In addition, they can throw other hormones, such as insulin, out of balance.

With that caution in mind, however, we are aware that there are times when you want to enjoy a special treat, a particularly favorite food that is high in saturated fats. On those occasions, you might find that pudding, ice cream, chocolate, and the like not only satisfy your pleasure centers, they can boost your levels of oxytocin as well.

*Vitamin C can chase away the blues
and make sex more desirable.*

You can get a similar oxytocin boost from the capsaicin in chile peppers and, as shown in research settings, by supplementation of vitamin C.

When it comes to raising your oxytocin levels, the Frustration-Induced Stress-Eater and the Quicky Stress-Eater have quite a bit in common. You share an excess of adrenaline and—by that hormone's action—a need for oxytocin. It's no surprise that you share a great many of the same recommendations as well.

So, if the thought that taking a vitamin could increase your desire for sex and decrease food cravings or the idea that eating spicy foods could help stop your stress-eating sounds intriguing, you'll find more essential information in The Quicky Stress-Eater's Cure (Chapter 39).

In addition, we suggest that you focus on giving yourself some exceptional "me" time: a chance to touch, to be touched as *you* desire, and, in doing so, to regain a most essential balance.

# 31

# The Social
# Stress-Eater's Cure

## YOUR PERSONALIZED PLAN

### Getting Started

The recommendations you find within this chapter have been individualized specifically for the Social Stress-Eater. To turn the Stress-Eating Cure Program into your personalized Stress-Eating Cure, simply apply these recommendations to the Stress-Eating Cure Program (Chapters 21 through 29).

In order to help Social Stress-Eaters eliminate their stress-eating and to lose weight, it would seem logical that they would need a personalized plan to help them decrease the levels of oxytocin that flow freely through their bodies. Scientific research, however, has shown that the opposite approach is far more effective.

If we start with the understanding that those things that give us true happiness and satisfaction in life are the very things that stimulate oxytocin release—which brings us a feeling of happiness and satisfaction— it seems impossible to imagine that the Social Stress-Eaters have too much of this good thing. Indeed, they do not.

We have found that the best way to bring hormonal balance back to the Social Stress-Eater is to focus on adrenaline levels instead. The greater problem is not that the Social Stress-Eater has too much oxytocin, but rather that they have too little adrenaline to help keep them motivated and focused on their eating and weight goals.

*You stress-eat when your own needs
get put on hold, too often, too long.*

By increasing adrenaline levels—just a little—by natural means, Social Stress-Eaters are able to find a better balance between concern for others and concern for self.

Before we offer suggestions on naturally increasing adrenaline, it's important to keep in mind *why* we are emphasizing that adrenaline levels should be raised to ideal levels and no higher and why they should be helped to rise naturally.

The negative effects of very high levels of adrenaline are well documented by scientists around the world. Extremely high levels of adrenaline have been tied to insulin resistance, cardiovascular problems, diabetes, and a plethora of other "diseases of civilization."[1] The effects of very low levels of the same hormone are less extensively studied. It does seem clear, however, that when it comes to adrenaline, Goldilocks had it on the nose: You want to go for "just right." And, of course, check with your doctor before making any changes to your diet or exercise regimen.

One of the easiest ways to bring balance to your adrenaline levels and regain focus on your eating and weight-loss goals is to simply take in a few quick, deep breaths. Breathe out quickly between each breath and inhale once again. Do this only a few times. You don't want to hyperventilate. Just as slow, deep breaths help you to relax, you will find that a few quick breaths taken in rapid succession can wake up your mind and body and pull you out of a daydreamlike mood.

Next time you find yourself slipping into a state of mindless eating, when you no longer seem to care whether you overeat or not, move to a place where you can be alone. Then imagine yourself as a prizefighter about to enter the ring.

Bounce from one foot to the other a bit, take a few quick breaths, and throw a punch or two. Your adrenaline levels will rise just a bit, and your ability to regain control of your eating will as well.

---

[1] Diseases of civilization are also called "lifestyle diseases." They can include, among others, atherosclerosis, cancer, type 2 diabetes, heart disease, metabolic syndrome, stroke, and obesity.

*If you want to keep the loving feeling*
*and increase your willpower too,*
*we've got some hot news for you.*

Another really helpful adrenaline raiser is found in some of the world's most delicious and spiciest meals. Capsaicin, found in chile peppers, is a powerful adrenaline booster.

Unless your preferences or medical concerns don't permit including chile pepper in some of your recipes or as a condiment served along with your favorite meal, some mild-to-moderate chile pepper might be just what you need to get the adrenaline juices flowing again.

Chile pepper has a surprising additional advantage as well. It is well known that most foods and activities that increase adrenaline decrease oxytocin at the same time. Our goal, as you know, is to keep the loving feeling that comes with high levels of oxytocin while bringing adrenaline levels into balance. Capsaicin and the hot chile peppers that contain it appear to do just that.

Though adrenaline levels rise with the consumption of foods containing hot chile pepper, oxytocin levels do as well! In that way, you can take part in the warm social experiences you enjoy while adding a bit of zip to your hormone equilibrium.

*There is a wonderful sign at Tokyo DisneySea.*
*It says, "Life is an astounding adventure."*
*For the Social Stress-Eater, that's the goal.*

One of the best ways we have found to bring adrenaline to an ideal level naturally and to keep it there is to focus on introducing new and exciting experiences in many different aspects of your life. As Japanese researcher Qing Li, MD, PhD, reported, "Adrenaline levels increase under circumstances of novelty, anticipation, unpredictability, and general emotional arousal." It makes sense that simple changes in your routine can help balance your adrenaline levels.

We suggest that you explore new and different ways of doing things and find novel, interesting things to do as you move through your day.

The changes do *not* need to be great; even small alterations in your daily habit can raise your energy levels.

Take a new route to the store, for example. A simple change in scenery may do you good and make you feel good at the same time. If you usually park in the same area of a parking lot, choose a new area. Stop in a store you would usually pass by. Smile at someone new. Give yourself a half hour a day to sample new things: Explore a new area of interest on the Internet, contact people you have wanted to connect with again (good for oxytocin and adrenaline levels at the same time), take a day trip or vacation to new places, or buy some new clothes (perhaps in a style that you've always wanted to wear). When it comes to your hormones, you may gain a lot by getting out of the comfortable but too-well-worn rut.

From this moment on, you'll do best if you keep in mind that your cure for Social Stress-Eating requires you to consider that your life is an adventure. Just the thought of all of the exciting opportunities that lie ahead has probably given you an adrenaline boost already! But the best is yet to come.

Give yourself real goals! Start out with one new activity each day; add another and another. Don't let negative judgments keep you from experiencing the thrill of feeling free and alive. As they say, don't knock it till you've tried it.

Once you've started your adventure, we think you'll find it more than rewarding on many levels. What a wonderful way to have fun, bring energy back into your life, and break free of Social Stress-Eating, all at the same time!

> *"Make it an adventure"* or
> *"Plan for pleasure."*
> *Which is it?*

In addition, we have found one other approach to Social Stress-Eating that is really effective: For all the balance that novelty brings, it works even better when it's combined with some smart planning—especially when you plan for pleasure.

Choose a new restaurant for novelty, for instance. But arrive early, before your friend(s), and look over the menu carefully. Or better yet, check out the restaurant's menu on the Internet. Decide what *you* want to eat before anyone arrives. Once your decision is made, don't discuss it. Be the first to order so that you are not influenced by the choices of others, and never, ever agree to share a dish. You are almost certain to end up getting too little or too much of the food you probably wouldn't have ordered in the first place. If you want it, order it. All for yourself. If you don't want to eat it all, enjoy the virtue of your own remarkable self-control.

Plan ahead for other ventures as well. If you know that the party you are about to attend may not have the food you need or like, eat something before you go. In that way, you are not at the mercy of those who are your hosts. You are not caught, yet again, in a situation that makes you choose between the needs of others and your own. If you're going to contribute to the food array, consider bringing food that *you* want to eat. That way, you can be sure of getting *exactly* what you want to eat.

*Social Stress-Eaters who exhibit a bit of healthy selfishness*
*are already on the road to success.*

If you don't feel comfortable eating fattening foods in front of others, but you want to enjoy the delicious foods that are part of your Stress-Eating Cure Program, pack your favorite goodies in your pocketbook or coat pocket and make your way to some place where you can enjoy them undisturbed.

Bathrooms can be perfect for a few moments of uninterrupted and well-earned indulgence. As an added bonus, just the excitement of taking care of your needs while maintaining your program ought to be enough to raise your adrenaline levels a bit! Best of all, you reap these wonderful benefits while you are having fun, bringing your body into balance, cutting your stress-hunger and cravings, breaking free of your stress-eating pattern, and losing weight!

# 32

# The Self-Sacrificing Stress-Eater's Cure

## Your Personalized Plan

### Getting Started

The recommendations you find within this chapter have been individualized specifically for the Self-Sacrificing Stress-Eater. To turn the Stress-Eating Cure Program into your personalized Stress-Eating Cure, simply apply these recommendations to the Stress-Eating Cure Program (Chapters 21 through 29).

As a Self-Sacrificing Stress-Eater, chances are you could do with some relief—and as quickly as possible. Your Stress-Eating Pattern is a sister disorder to the Frustration-Induced Stress-Eater. You both have high levels of adrenaline. But, in contrast to the Frustration-Induced Stress-Eater who has low levels of the bonding hormone, oxytocin, you have low levels of the pleasure hormone, dopamine.

That singular difference is very important. It paves the way for you to be able to experience more pleasure in your life—quickly!

Remember, before you can effectively increase your dopamine levels (and the pleasure dopamine brings), it is important to lower your levels of adrenaline.

Fortunately, there are lots of ways of decreasing adrenaline levels, some quite surprising. You may have heard that to decrease adrenaline levels you must meditate, become tranquil in mind and body, and enter a Zenlike state. Indeed, meditation works for many people, but it does little good if you fail to recognize the adrenaline-makers that you're putting in your mouth!

*Some of the foods you love don't love you. But there are ways to deal with these tempting troublemakers!*

Diet drinks (caffeinated and decaf), mustard, chile peppers, even cinnamon can raise your adrenaline levels (which may be why they're so enjoyable!). Highly palatable foods (those that are particularly delicious) can act as adrenaline-spikers as well.

Before we go any further, please understand that no one expects you to give up these delightful treats. Instead, you will learn to balance them to limit their impact on adrenaline levels.

When it comes to spicy foods, for example, be sure to eat them with stomach-coating creamy foods. There is a reason that spicy Mexican food is often served with a big dollop of sour cream on the side or that fiery Indian food is often served alongside a wonderful yogurt-cucumber dip called *raita*. People around the world have learned that a creamy balance to hot and spicy flavors is essential to the well-being of the body.

Before you reach for a spicy condiment to add flavor to your food or you get ready to dig into a wonderfully spicy dish, make sure you have a creamy, soothing dish as well. Start the meal off with the creamier food and bring on the big guns a bit later.

*You can have your cake and eat it, too.*
*You just have to know when to eat it.*

Here's some more good news: You *can* enjoy highly palatable foods while limiting their adrenaline-revving potential. The best way to enjoy extraordinarily tasty foods without throwing your hormonal balance out of kilter is to include these foods in your daily Big Balanced Breakfast or Alternative Meal.[1]

---

[1] The Alternative Meal is a daily, balanced meal that replaces the Big Balanced Breakfast. It may be eaten at any time later in the day or evening. In combination with Balancing Foods, it should always contain a good portion of Comfort Foods (pages 248–51).

When you eat especially flavorful foods only once a day, your body will be better equipped to handle the rush of hormones than if these foods were encountered regularly throughout the day. For your other meals, stick to pleasure-giving foods that fill you and please you but are more familiar (and, so, less stimulating).

Diet drinks fall into the same category as highly palatable foods. If you must have them, try to include them in your Big Balanced Breakfast or Alternative Meal only. If you can do without sugar substitutes completely, do yourself a favor and let them go. You'll find important information on these powerful hormone disruptors in Chapter 41, Stress-Eating Busters. We suggest that you take a moment and read about them right now.

In any case, remember that if you *must* have sugar substitutes, have them as infrequently as possible, always with food, and preferably at your Big Balanced Breakfast or Alternative Meal.

As you know, the hormonal imbalance that sets off stress-hunger, cravings, stress-eating, and weight gain in the Self-Sacrificing Stress-Eater is similar in many ways to that of the Frustration-Induced Stress-Eater (with the exception that the Self-Sacrificing Stress-Eater's hormonal imbalance may have persisted for a longer time). It is no surprise, then, that many of the Self-Sacrificing Stress-Eater's recommendations will be similar to those suggested for the Frustration-Induced Stress-Eater, as well.

Look over all of the personalized recommendations aimed at balancing adrenaline levels on pages 183–85. Though they describe changes that will reduce stress-hunger, cravings, stress-eating, and weight problems for the Frustration-Induced Stress-Eater, they can do wonders for the Self-Sacrificing Stress-Eater as well.

*As your adrenaline levels begin to balance out,*
*your capacity for joy will return naturally!*

Your adrenaline levels will begin to find a natural balance, and you will find that simple daily activities will once again bring you pleasure. Make time for your own experiences of joy. They are your rightful reward.

# 33

# The Secret
# Stress-Eater's Cure

## Your Personalized Plan

### Getting Started

The recommendations you find within this chapter have been individualized specifically for the Secret Stress-Eater. To turn the Stress-Eating Cure Program into your personalized Stress-Eating Cure, simply apply these recommendations to the Stress-Eating Cure Program (Chapters 21 through 29).

To help put an end to their stress-hunger, cravings, stress-eating, and weight gain, Secret Stress-Eaters need a personalized plan designed to decrease the high levels of adrenaline and insulin that drive their cycle of secret eating.

Any act of Secret Stress-Eating, especially when there exists the possibility of being discovered—either immediately or in the long run— is almost certain to lead to great spikes in adrenaline levels. Surprisingly, our first recommendation to the Secret Stress-Eater is *not* necessarily to bring your eating out in the open, however. Nor do we recommend that you make a confession of your past behaviors. If, indeed, either of these choices feels *right* to you and you are absolutely ready to do so, then we would encourage you, as always, to do that which appears in your best interest. Before you take any action, be certain that you are not setting yourself up for an emotional confrontation that would offer a ready-made reason to return to Secret Stress-Eating.

*Your eating, your weight, your hopes, and your dreams*
*do not have to be the stuff of light conversation.*

Rather than suddenly bringing your Secret Stress-Eating behavior out into the open or trying to make everyone understand what it's like to experience intense hunger and cravings as you do, we suggest that you begin to enjoy the foods that are part of your Stress-Eating Cure Program with a trusted friend. If you really need to, you might explain the program and share with that person the reason that you include your favorite foods in your Big Balanced Breakfast or Alternative Meal.[1] If you would rather *not* go into an explanation (which would be our suggestion), then you might simply say, "I'm trying a little experiment for now. I'll tell you all about it when I see how it works out."

This latter response puts your eating into a no-big-deal category (after all, who can argue with a little experiment?). What's more, you've succeeded at putting off a conversation that neither you nor your friend really wanted to pursue.

After your weight loss has become obvious, you still have the option of not discussing the matter. Simply say that you are still learning about this way of eating and that you'll give more details when you're sure you won't be gaining the weight back.

*If a trusted friend pushes you to talk about something*
*you'd rather not discuss, then maybe he/she isn't*
*such a good friend after all.*

If your friend pushes you to discuss the matter, we urge you to hold your ground. Then choose another, less pushy person with whom to break your Secret Stress-Eating Pattern.

In time, as you begin to lose weight, you'll feel more comfortable eating your Comfort Foods in the company of others. Most important, and we say this with great joy, as you begin to find your hormonal balance, your feelings of trust, understanding, and connection will

---

[1] The Alternative Meal is a daily, balanced meal that replaces the Big Balanced Breakfast. It may be eaten at any time later in the day or evening. In combination with Balancing Foods, it should always contain a good portion of Comfort Foods (pages 248–51).

return. And so will your personal power. Those who deserve your trust will experience it once again. Those who would judge or condemn you will see that you cannot be intimidated or shamed.

You will recover the ability to come out of the shadows and to claim the same rights as anyone to respect, to unconditional love, and to life's basic pleasures—including the food you truly love—to be enjoyed and savored without judgment, shame, or blame.

## Shared Suggestions, Unique Help

High adrenaline levels are not unique to Secret Stress-Eaters. This hormonal imbalance is experienced by Frustration-Induced Stress-Eaters and Self-Sacrificing Stress-Eaters as well.[2] In each of the chapters devoted to recommendations for the Frustration-Induced Stress-Eater and the Self-Sacrificing Stress-Eater, you'll find suggestions that can be of particular value to you as well. In Chapter 30, The Frustration-Induced Stress-Eater's Cure, you'll find remarkably pleasurable experiences that will help lower your adrenaline levels by raising oxytocin levels. In Chapter 32, The Self-Sacrificing Stress-Eater's Cure, you'll discover which foods and drinks may be spiking your adrenaline levels and how to easily limit their impact.

The Secret Stress-Eater's high insulin levels are experienced by Carbohydrate-Induced Stress-Eaters and others as well. Chapter 34, The Carbohydrate-Induced Stress-Eater's Cure, will offer you a wide variety of suggestions designed to bring your high insulin levels back into balance quickly and easily.

Read these three chapters. Although they are not written specifically for you, you'll find many surprising, effective, and enjoyable adrenaline-reducing suggestions.

---

[2] In each of their respective cases, high levels of adrenaline are combined with other, distinct hormonal imbalances.

# 34

# The
# Carbohydrate-Induced
# Stress-Eater's Cure

## YOUR PERSONALIZED PLAN

### Getting Started

The recommendations you find within this chapter have been individualized specifically for the Carbohydrate-Induced Stress-Eater. To turn the Stress-Eating Cure Program into your personalized Stress-Eating Cure, simply apply these recommendations to the Stress-Eating Cure Program (Chapters 21 through 29).

In an attempt to break free of the power that carbohydrate-rich foods can have over their eating and their weight, many Carbohydrate-Induced Stress-Eaters have tried to follow low-carb weight-loss programs.

At first, most Carbohydrate-Induced Stress-Eaters experience a remarkable freedom from cravings and a rapid weight loss on these programs. The problem, of course, is that no low-carbohydrate diet can be followed for a prolonged period of time. Dieters who try to do so will either get sick and tired of the limitations of the program or they will just get sick.

To try to avoid both problems, some low-carb diet gurus have invented subsequent stages in which greater and greater quantities of carbohydrate-rich foods are added to the diet. Indeed, adding carbohydrates does meet the need for including carbohydrates in the Carbohydrate-Induced Stress-Eaters diet. The problem, however—and it's a major one—is that on low-carb programs, as you add carbohydrate-rich food to the eating program, the cravings, hunger, and weight gain return.

It may look as if there is no way around the problem. Carbohydrates are needed to sustain life,[1] but when you eat them, you can't stop.

There is, however, a struggle-free solution to the Carbohydrate-Induced Stress-Eater's dilemma. The Stress-Eating Cure Program will supply your body with the carbohydrates it needs every day in the foods you love and that bring you comfort. By using your individual hormonal chemistry to maximize the program's effectiveness and, at the same time, using your hormonal rhythms each day to maximize your weight loss, you will be able to disarm your body's resistance to weight loss and break free of stress-hunger and cravings.

*Add, don't restrict. Balance, don't eliminate.*
*And enjoy it, all the way.*

The answer may seem counterintuitive, but sometimes you need to add foods to your eating program rather than further restrict them, balance a food rather than eliminate it, and enjoy a delicious, satisfying breakfast that will sustain you throughout the day rather than force yourself to run on empty.

We know that you've tried to lose weight the hard way. We also know that while your strong-arm attempts worked for a while, in the end they failed. Now, it may be time to take the pain, strain, and stress out of your eating and weight-loss program and give your body exactly what it has so desperately needed for so long.

When you first experienced the beginnings of Carbohydrate-Induced Stress-Eating, it is likely that you found yourself favoring starches and sweet foods. Chances are, your meals contained a great

---

[1] Carbohydrate-rich foods are essential to good health and must be included in every Carbohydrate-Induced Stress-Eater's eating program. Reducing the frequency with which carbohydrate-rich foods are eaten has been shown to lead to less hunger and fewer cravings and greater weight loss than that experienced on a low-carbohydrate diet.

proportion of pasta, bread, potatoes, and—depending on the severity of your insulin imbalance—dessert as well. A short time after completing a meal, you probably were back in the kitchen looking for something to munch on or for some sweet treat.

*Carbohydrate-Induced Stress-Eaters*
*prefer a table full of appetizers*
*to a traditional full, balanced meal.*

During later stages of Carbohydrate-Induced Stress-Eating, however, preferences for starches, snack food, sweets, and junk food take hold and crowd out almost all desire for balanced meals. In this stage, it is likely you will subsist mainly on fast food, sandwiches, snack foods, and sweets. You may rarely, if ever, cook for yourself. Even the thought of a good, balanced meal may offer little, if any, appeal.

These are the signs that your body is releasing greater insulin rushes and that your body is becoming resistant to this hormone overload.

If you find that you tend to skip breakfast on a frequent basis; if fast food, junk food, snacks, or sweets have become part of your nutritional norm; if your balanced, home-cooked, sit-down-at-a-plate-and-eat-at-home meals have sort of fallen by the wayside, we recommend that you follow the Quick-Start Plan of the program. Start with Chapter 22, then continue on to Chapter 23.

The Quick-Start Plan has been designed to cut your stress-hunger, cravings, and stress-eating in a matter of a few days and help you to begin taking off the pounds quickly. Most important, it is a fast track to getting those insulin levels back into balance.

*Skipping breakfast? You'll never guess*
*who is telling you not to eat!*

One of the two most success-sabotaging behaviors of Carbohydrate-Induced Stress-Eaters is their tendency to skip breakfast. Most Carbohydrate-Induced Stress-Eaters simply have little, if any, need to eat in the morning.

Ironically, researchers have shown that skipping breakfast is one of the greatest errors a Carbohydrate-Induced Stress-Eater can make. While they are concentrating on what they think they *shouldn't* be eating, they're losing sight of the foods and meals that they *should* be eating.

"But I was *so* good," Carbohydrate-Induced Stress-Eaters will exclaim. "I ate almost nothing!" And that, we have to tell them, may have been one of their biggest mistakes.

You will discover some amazing scientific findings about the importance of breakfast in the correction of hormonally induced eating and weight gain in Chapter 23, The Big Breakfast Breakthrough.

These findings confirm that eating a Big Balanced Breakfast followed by balanced meals (that do not stimulate hormonal imbalances) is clearly the best way to lose weight and to keep it off without struggle, cravings, or sacrifice.

Even though a greater amount of food is eaten throughout the day, if you start your morning with a good, balanced breakfast, you will see that you are likely to lose up to *five times* the weight that you would on low-carbohydrate, restrictive diets.

If your insulin levels are high, you might not feel like eating breakfast. This is insulin's way of keeping you hooked on the carbs. Your body has learned that if you don't eat breakfast, you're more likely to reach for starches, snack foods, junk foods, and sweets later in the day.

After a few days of balanced meals and your insulin levels beginning to return to normal, however, you'll begin looking forward to the delight of a Big Balanced Breakfast to start your day.[2] Best of all, you'll find it gives you all of the punch and the pleasure that only junk food used to supply.

*Think sugar substitutes are keeping off the pounds?*
*They're doing just the opposite.*

The second success-sabotaging mistake that most Carbohydrate-Induced Stress-Eaters make is relying on sugar substitutes. Now, before

---

[2] For stress-eaters who do not wish to or cannot include a Big Balanced Breakfast in their program, Alternative Meals can be substituted. The Alternative Meal is a daily, balanced meal that replaces the Big Balanced Breakfast. It may be eaten at any time later in the day or evening. In combination with Balancing Foods, it should always contain a good portion of Comfort Foods (pages 248–51).

we begin, no one is going to tell you that you *have* to give up your sugar substitute (either artificial sweetener or "natural" sweetener). We simply want you to consider what scientists have discovered about the power of these sweeteners to raise your insulin levels and keep you in a carbohydrate addiction cycle.

Read over the recommendations on page 228. You will find many choices. You might decide to continue your use of sugar substitutes while using our suggestions to help balance the sweeteners' effects on your insulin balance.

Or you might choose to limit your use of these sweeteners or give them up altogether by using our tested recommendations that make breaking free of them far easier than you might imagine. In any case, keep your mind open to the possibility that sugar substitutes may be fueling your Carbohydrate-Induced Stress-Eating and, at the same time, doubling your chances for adult-onset diabetes.

If sugar substitutes have no pull for you, terrific! If they do, however, be sure to read the appropriate section in Chapter 41, Stress-Eating Busters.

*Think that exercise burns calories?*
*Not enough to make a bit of difference.*
*But it does something far more helpful*
*to your weight loss!*

When it comes to cutting your cravings and losing weight, making time for some activity in your life can be really helpful. Here's the surprising part: It's not the food energy that exercise requires that makes you lose weight! The number of calories burned during activity makes up a very tiny part of the calories you use up just staying alive. You'd need 6 to 7 hours of a strenuous workout to lose 1 pound (which you would probably gain back from the protein bar that you ate on your way out of the gym).

The reason that exercise is important for weight loss (and for health), especially to the Carbohydrate-Induced Stress-Eater, is that moderate exercise helps bring insulin levels back into balance. More balanced insulin levels mean fewer cravings, less of a tendency to store food energy as fat, and a normal cycle of taking in food and then burning calories.

*Too much exercise can be just as bad, even worse,*
*than none at all.*

Excessive exercise rather than moderate activity can have a negative effect on the body. Too much of a good thing, even exercise, can stress the body and raise cortisol, adrenaline, and insulin levels—a state of affairs you want to avoid if at all possible.

So, for now, unless otherwise directed by your physician, stick with a mild or moderate exercise regimen.

While moderate exercise or activity alone is unlikely to pull you out of a Carbohydrate-Induced Stress-Eating Cycle, when it is included as part of the Stress-Eating Cure Program itself, it can help bring your body back into a hunger-free, craving-free balance.

Remember that your hormones can work for you just as easily as they can sometimes work against you. It's not your body you need to fight but, rather, the old rules that have repeatedly failed you in the past. You have a whole new future ahead of you now.

# 35

# The Anxiety-Induced
# Stress-Eater's Cure

## YOUR PERSONALIZED PLAN

### Getting Started

The recommendations you find within this chapter have been individualized specifically for the Anxiety-Induced Stress-Eater. To turn the Stress-Eating Cure Program into your personalized Stress-Eating Cure, simply apply these recommendations to the Stress-Eating Cure Program (Chapters 21 through 29).

The same hormonal imbalance that fuels your cravings, stress-hunger, stress-eating, and weight gain can also make you a strongly motivated achiever. Anxiety-Induced Stress-Eaters often prefer the Quick-Start Plan of the program.

When deciding between the Step-by-Step Plan and the Quick-Start Plan, consider that the Quick-Start Plan is most likely to cut your cravings and hunger within a few days and start taking off the pounds quickly.

*For you, in particular, it's essential to move at your own pace.*

If you choose the easier-paced Step-by-Step Plan, move through the six steps as quickly as you desire.

Be certain, however, that you understand each of the steps and that you have made the recommended changes before you move to the next step. You may have a tendency to either hold back for fear of making a mistake or rush forward (perhaps for the same reason).

When choosing your Comfort Foods, it's a good idea to select those that require chewing. As a general rule of thumb, the less-sweet cakes and cookies are usually a better choice than candy for all stress-eaters. On the other hand, if candy is one of the several Comfort Foods you choose, you may find that chewy candies such as taffy, licorice, or similar sweets offer the most satisfaction.

*Frozen candy bars: a perfect Comfort Food treat*
*for your Stress-Eating Pattern.*

If you desire a candy bar such as Snickers or Three Musketeers as one of your Comfort Food choices, it's a good idea to freeze the candy bar first and then break it into bite-size pieces. The frozen bits of candy bar will require a great deal more chewing effort than softer chocolate bars that seem to slip down your throat unnoticed. Just one precaution: Don't freeze the candy so hard that you could harm a tooth!

For your Balancing Proteins and Balancing Vegetables and Salads, be sure to include lots of natural foods. Lean steak or spare ribs and crunchy vegetables including celery and green peppers or green beans require a great deal of biting and chewing. These foods give you something that, literally, you can tear into. They provide a great outlet for the excess of stress hormones that have been driving you to eat too quickly, too often, or too much.

*Chewy, crunchy foods can offer you special satisfaction.*

Nuts and seeds are a good choice for you, with whole pumpkin seeds and sunflower seeds at the top of the list. Whenever possible, choose nuts and seeds with shells rather than the shelled varieties. Nuts or seeds in the shell require a bit of work for the prize. If the shells don't slow you down, your hormones could drive you to consume great quantities of nuts or seeds before you know it.

If possible, your Stress-Eating Busters (Chapter 41) should center around physical activity, fast-moving and full-body workouts. It is likely that your hormone levels will not respond as well to slow-moving or deep-breathing stress-reduction techniques. It's a good idea to use up the energy and, in doing so, bring the excess cortisol and adrenaline levels into balance naturally. Be careful not to engage in so much physical activity that it, too, throws your hormonal balance out of kilter.

Kickboxing, dancing with a strong, fast beat, jumping rope, jogging, and calisthenics can all offer an excellent boost to balancing your hormones.

On the other hand, if you just don't have it in you to undertake a rigorous workout or such vigorous activity is unwise for you, choose a lighter activity such as walking or dancing (you can even do this alone in your room), if only for 10 minutes a day. After your hormones return to balance and your energy kicks in, you may move to higher levels of activity naturally. If not, just continue the activities you've chosen.

Meditation, tai chi, and other sedentary or slow-moving relaxation methods may actually worsen an Anxiety-Induced Stress-Eater's hormonal imbalance. You may find that they make you anxious about being anxious. Unless you really desire to do so, we wouldn't recommend these activities as a balancing option for the Anxiety-Induced Stress-Eater—at least not for now.

*Sex, masturbation, and massage can help bring your body back into balance . . . quickly!*

Sex and masturbation appear to be excellent means of balancing an Anxiety-Induced Stress-Eater's hormones! Oxytocin, the bonding hormone released after sex or masturbation, suppresses adrenaline. And just imagine, you'll be giving yourself pleasure for the sake of your weight-loss program!

For the Anxiety-Induced Stress-Eater, one of the most powerful Stress-Eating Busters for cutting stress-hunger, cravings, and stress-eating and for increasing weight loss is massage. In several studies at the

University of Miami School of Medicine, reported by Tiffany Field, PhD, and her colleagues in the *International Journal of Neuroscience*, massage was found to have a powerful influence on cortisol levels.

A wide and varied population was tested, including people suffering from depression, sexual abuse, anorexia or bulimia, asthma, chronic fatigue, HIV, job stress, activity stress, high blood pressure, chronic pain, and those dealing with the stresses of getting older. All showed remarkably reduced levels of cortisol following massage.

Though the period of massage was, in some cases, only 15 minutes long, twice a week, and delivered in a chair, cortisol levels were reduced by as much as 45 percent!

Thousands of other researchers report similar findings along with added benefits to health and well-being. Our professional and personal experiences confirm these findings as well.

If you don't have the money for a professional massage, find a friend to exchange a good backrub with or ask your mate for some special time. Just two times a week ought to do it.

When it comes to massage, however, you don't necessarily need anyone else to help you lower your cortisol levels! Maria Hernandez-Reif, PhD, and her colleagues discovered that a 5-minute self-massage of the hand or ear three times a day had remarkable results. Among their subjects—who were attempting to quit smoking—anxiety levels dropped by 25 percent, the intensity of cravings for cigarettes dropped by 40 percent, and the number of cigarettes smoked dropped by 30 percent . . . naturally, without struggle, simply by adding a few minutes of self-massage each day.

*You've been balancing your hormones all along without knowing it!*

Chances are, there have been times when you found yourself massaging your neck or rubbing your face when you truly needed to lower the stress level you were experiencing.

It's remarkable to think that you might have been attempting to bring down your cortisol levels without even knowing it! Clearly, for the

Anxiety-Induced Stress-Eater, massage is an important Stress-Eating Buster to consider.

*Five minutes!*
*That's all it takes to lower your stress hormones.*
*And you can do it anywhere!*

In our own research, we have seen the power of tiny breaks of self-massage in action as well. Just a few minutes of self-massage applied to the feet, neck, wrists, and face can improve body chemistry remarkably. For the Anxiety-Induced Stress-Eater, in particular, touch, either physical or emotional, can help restore a much-needed balance.

Now, you might give lip service to the fact that, indeed, you will take the time to employ one or more of the recommendations that we offer; but when it comes to taking action, you tell yourself that you just don't have the time. If you should find yourself in just such an internal conversation, we ask you to imagine a child or pet for whom you have affection. Consider that for some reason that child or pet is filled with fear. Wouldn't you give at least 5 minutes of your time to stroke and comfort it, to have it understand that it is safe, and to feel it relax in your arms? Well, then, are you not worth that same kind of comforting and care?

# 36

# The Task-Avoiding
# Stress-Eater's Cure

## YOUR PERSONALIZED PLAN

### Getting Started

The recommendations you find within this chapter have been individualized specifically for the Task-Avoiding Stress-Eater. To turn the Stress-Eating Cure Program into your personalized Stress-Eating Cure, simply apply these recommendations to the Stress-Eating Cure Program (Chapters 21 through 29).

The first task of the Task-Avoiding Stress-Eater's Cure is to bring their cortisol and dopamine levels back into balance. The Stress-Eating Cure Program will help bring these hormones back into equilibrium naturally. We would suggest, however, that you move through the program in a way that is unique to your needs.

Throughout the program, you will be given choices. At first, you will be asked to choose between the Step-by-Step Plan and the Quick-Start Plan of the Stress-Eating Cure Program. Later, you will freely select the foods you prefer and the Stress-Eating Busters to enhance your hormone-balancing food choices.

As you make each of these choices, consider this rhyme:

> *Baby steps will get you there,*
> *no push, demand, or blame,*
> *Change one small thing, one at a time,*
> *that's how to win the game.*

Although the challenges that a Task-Avoiding Stress-Eater faces are no game, the simple poem may "rhyme-mind" you to take it easy and slow.

> *Your hormones are already yelling at you!*
> *You don't need a chorus of blame.*

Remember, as a Task-Avoiding Stress-Eater, when you face overwhelming demands, your body produces too much cortisol and too little oxytocin. Low levels of oxytocin (the bonding hormone) are almost certain to lead to high levels of adrenaline. With high levels of the two major stress hormones, adrenaline and cortisol, surging through your body, the last thing you need is even more pressure.

Although there may be times that even Task-Avoiding Stress-Eaters could use a bit of a kick in the pants for just not *wanting* to face some task or complete some chore, in general, if you are feeling anxious about a challenge, break it down into manageable pieces.

There is an old joke that asks: "How do you eat an elephant?" The answer: "One bite at a time!"

In the same way, the greatest of all tasks can be tackled one subtask at a time. Each small task that you complete will make it easier to accomplish the next and so on.

Although the thought of deadlines may make you cringe, we urge you to consider this: When you combine a series of small-step changes with a generous deadline, you are far more likely to be successful.

If someone asked you to run up a twenty-story staircase, chances are they'd find you panting and exhausted somewhere along the way (that's assuming you even considered undertaking such a task). On the other hand, if you were requested to ascend one step at a time for some considerable compensation, and if there were a comfortable place to rest along the way, the job would be quite doable.

> *Task-Avoiding Stress-Eaters should reward themselves*
> *often and generously.*

This last point brings up another important factor to your success.

As a Task-Avoiding Stress-Eater, you must, must, *must* reward yourself for your achievements. Rewards help reduce anxiety and reinforce the experience of success. Besides, you have it coming!

So, for each accomplishment on the program, give yourself a reward. Say, for example, you've added a salad to your midafternoon snack as per Step #3 of the program. Terrific! Now, make sure you get that special dressing you really like. Or, if finances allow, purchase the DVD of the latest season of your favorite TV show as part of the Stress-Eating Busters recommendations (see Chapter 41).

No money? No worry! Take a bit of personal time for reading or listening to music or luxuriate in a hot bath. Whatever the pleasure, it matters little as long as you remember that you've earned it, one small step at a time.

In the end, you'll find you've climbed to the top of the staircase; and, what's more, you'll discover that you've enjoyed yourself all along the way.

# 37

# The Guilt-Induced
# Stress-Eater's Cure

## YOUR PERSONALIZED PLAN

### Getting Started

The recommendations you find within this chapter have been individualized specifically for the Guilt-Induced Stress-Eater. To turn the Stress-Eating Cure Program into your personalized Stress-Eating Cure, simply apply these recommendations to the Stress-Eating Cure Program (Chapters 21 through 29).

As a Guilt-Induced Stress-Eater, your focus is simple and straightforward: Cut the cause of your hormonal imbalance and break the cycle. Rather than focus on reducing oxytocin and the wonderful feelings of connection and affection it engenders, it makes more sense to focus on insulin, the real villain in the Guilt-Induced Stress-Eater's hormonal imbalance.

As you begin the Stress-Eating Cure Program, we suggest that you try the Quick-Start Plan. The fast-paced change it offers will help you balance your insulin levels, cut your stress-hunger and cravings, clear your thinking, and help free you from your Stress-Eating Cycle without delay.

After you've read over the basics of the program (Chapter 21) and details on the Quick-Start Plan (Chapter 22), if you still prefer to start with the Step-by-Step Plan, that's okay. We want to make certain that you familiarize yourself with your choice before you begin. The Step-by-Step

Plan may take you an extra week or two to get the same results, but both plans will deliver the same results.

*Three simple strategies combine their power to free you*
*from stress-eating—quickly and for good!*

With the program guidelines in place, three essential strategies should help ensure your success on the program by combating your high levels of insulin.

The first and second of these strategies entail countering Comfort-Food Act-Alikes that could easily sabotage the success of your Stress-Eating Cure Program. Given your hormonal imbalance, it is likely that you are particularly vulnerable to the effects of sugar substitutes as well as to glutamates.

You will learn more about these two villains in detail in Chapter 41, which is devoted entirely to Stress-Eating Busters. The information you'll find in that chapter will provide the best personalized recommendations we could offer for your pattern of stress-eating.

Read the Stress-Eating Buster pages carefully. They hold information that will be essential to your success.

The third strategy to help ensure that insulin levels remain under control involves a healthy serving of physical activity, in particular, fast-moving and full-body workouts.

It is unlikely that your high levels of insulin will respond well to slow-moving activities such as tai chi or the deep-breathing techniques practiced in meditation. For your particular high-insulin, high-oxytocin hormone pattern, a couple of good bouts of jumping rope, vigorous dancing, or jogging might be a better choice.

On the other hand, be careful not to engage in so much physical activity that it, too, throws your hormonal balance out of kilter.

If you just don't have it in you to undertake a rigorous workout or if such vigorous activity is unwise for you, choose a less-demanding activity such as walking or dancing to a moderate beat, if only for 10 minutes a day.

After your hormones return to balance and your energy kicks in, you may move to higher levels of activity naturally. If not, just continue the activities you've chosen.

In combination, the reduction or elimination of Comfort Food Act-Alikes and a modest yet regular exercise regimen should help to bring hormone levels into equilibrium.

One word of warning: Do not begin to incorporate the three essential strategies above until you have moved through each of the six steps of the Step-by-Step Plan and feel that you have the program well in hand. After your eating program is in place, however, you are free to add the three essential strategies to your program and watch as each helps you shed both the guilt and the pounds at the same time.

# 38

# The Exhaustion-Induced Stress-Eater's Cure

## YOUR PERSONALIZED PLAN

### Getting Started

The recommendations you find within this chapter have been individualized specifically for the Exhaustion-Induced Stress-Eater. To turn the Stress-Eating Cure Program into your personalized Stress-Eating Cure, simply apply these recommendations to the Stress-Eating Cure Program (Chapters 21 through 29). As an Exhaustion-Induced Stress-Eater, it is tempting to fall into a pattern of inaction. You may tell yourself that you'll just give it time and wait for yourself to pull out of it. The thought of starting a new program or a new way of life may seem overwhelming.

You may have moments of fantasy in which you can easily imagine all that you would love to change in your life, but when it comes to taking action, you find that you simply don't have the time, energy, motivation, or all of the above. If you think we're going to tell you to buck up, make some drastic change, and make it fast, you're in for a surprise!

*You've pushed yourself far too hard for far too long.*

When Exhaustion-Induced Stress-Eaters push themselves too hard to lose weight too quickly, their exhaustion may actually worsen. Their cravings may increase in intensity and frequency, and they may find it more difficult than ever to lose weight. The best rule of thumb for the Exhaustion-Induced Stress-Eater is to move slowly, in small steps, and, most important, at a comfortable pace.

A guideline you will find in the Stress-Eating Cure Program recommends that you add some Balancing Foods to your lunch and after 2 days add the same to your dinner. But consider that, for you, it might be best to make the first change and continue to incorporate that change into your daily eating plan for as long as you need before moving on to the next change. Certainly, you don't want to lose momentum. It is true that the more quickly you bring your hormones back into balance, the more quickly your stress-hunger, cravings, stress-eating, and weight problems will become fading memories. On the other hand, for you, in particular, it's important to find your right pacing.

Listening to your own timing may be a learning experience at first. It is likely that you are used to doing things in an all-or-nothing manner. It can be a good opportunity to get in touch with *your* needs, however, and to experience and trust what's right for you.

When you decide between the Step-by-Step Plan and the Quick-Start Plan, we believe that the Step-by-Step Plan is most likely to give you the results you want without the rebound it is always best to avoid.

As you begin to add Balancing Foods and Comfort Foods into your eating plan, you may find that you have little desire to cook for yourself or make the effort to plan your meals. You'll find tempting, easy recipes made for just such a lack of enthusiasm and special recommendations in a chapter devoted to Stress-Eating Busters (Chapter 41). Read over these sections carefully. They will help you get the food you need and the pleasure you want without very much effort at all.

Be certain that you pay attention to balancing your Big Balanced Breakfast and Alternative Meals.[1] Your eating pattern can make it easy for you to "carbo drift"; that is, begin to eat greater and greater quantities of Comfort Foods and smaller and smaller quantities of Balancing Foods in these meals.

---

[1] The Alternative Meal is a daily, balanced meal that replaces the Big Balanced Breakfast. It may be eaten at any time later in the day or evening. In combination with Balancing Foods, it should always contain a good portion of Comfort Foods (pages 248–51).

When you choose your Hormone-Balancing Activities in the Stress-Eating Busters chapter, start slowly with only a few minutes of walking or exercise and work up to longer workout times. For you, it would be better to exercise at a good pace for a shorter period of time rather than participate in a more leisurely activity for a longer period of time.

Dancing with a strong, fast beat, jumping rope, jogging, and calisthenics are excellent hormone-balancing activities. If, however, you are not about to undertake a rigorous workout, choose a lighter activity such as walking or moving easily to a song you enjoy, if only for 10 minutes a day. After your hormones return to balance and your energy kicks in, you may move to higher levels of activity naturally. If not, just continue the activities you've chosen. As always, check with your physician before making any exercise or activity choice.

*Let the warmth spread through you and rejuvenate you.*

Include warm beverages at the end of your meals whenever possible. You will probably find that a warm cup of tea or coffee (regular or decaffeinated, as appropriate) hits the spot and makes you feel that the meal is complete. For the most satisfaction, take time to sit and enjoy it.

Meditation, tai chi, and other sedentary or slow-moving relaxation methods that do not progress to more rigorous activity are not the best first choice for Exhaustion-Induced Stress-Eaters (unless otherwise indicated). Getting yourself up and moving may be one of the best things you can do to bring your hormones back into balance.

Most of all, keep focused on your needs, your preferences, your timing. Finally, it's your turn. It's been a long time coming.

# 39

# The Quicky
# Stress-Eater's Cure

## YOUR PERSONALIZED PLAN

### Getting Started

The recommendations you find within this chapter have been individualized specifically for the Quicky Stress-Eater. To turn the Stress-Eating Cure Program into your personalized Stress-Eating Cure, simply apply these recommendations to the Stress-Eating Cure Program (Chapters 21 through 29).

As a Quicky Stress-Eater, the main focus of your personalized plan will be to decrease the levels of adrenaline that may be flooding your body. You can do that best by boosting levels of the bonding hormone, oxytocin.

The Stress-Eating Cure Program, either the Step-by-Step Plan or the Quick-Start Plan, can help you balance one hormone by balancing the other. For the Quicky Stress-Eater, it is important to bring down high levels of adrenaline as quickly as possible while not causing a hormonal rebound at the same time.

Combining the eating portion of the Stress-Eating Cure Program with Stress-Eating Busters (Chapter 41) can offer you relief and pleasure, and it should put you well on the way to raising your oxytocin levels and lowering adrenaline levels as well.

*One of the best ways to bring your adrenaline in line
is going to surprise you.*

In addition, physical contact with someone you feel connected to (whether platonic or sexual in nature), massage, self-massage, and masturbation are most likely to raise your oxytocin levels. If not sexual, then the more sensual the experience, the better. Wrap yourself in your favorite blanket, brush your hair, get a good back scratch—they can all help to bring your hormone levels back into balance.

*What do chocolate and your pet have in common?*
*Both make you feel good because they can affect the same hormones.*

Emotionally satisfying experiences that do not involve physical contact can raise oxytocin levels as well. Taking the time to enjoy some private time with a special friend, petting your dog or stroking your cat, being empathetic toward a stranger, performing a simple act of kindness, sharing a conversation over a satisfying meal, listening to your favorite CD (over and over), singing, playing a musical instrument, breathing in deeply pleasurable and reminiscent smells, watching a sunrise or sunset, sitting and watching the ocean, or just sitting and holding hands with someone you love—all can do their part in raising your oxytocin levels. And raising oxytocin will help lower your adrenaline in some of the most enjoyable ways imaginable.

Being with a loved pet, even *without* the physical connection of petting, has also been shown to raise oxytocin levels. Indeed, being with a beloved pet can be as effective as talking with a friend or family member. Scientists have proven that people with pets tend to live (and love) longer. Perhaps the higher levels of oxytocin and lower levels of adrenaline are the reason!

The Balancing Foods and Comfort Foods that you enjoy as part of your program can have a great effect on your levels of oxytocin. Fatty foods release far more oxytocin than most other foods. That's one of the reasons why so many people find rich, high-fat, smooth, and creamy foods so satisfying. Please note that we are *not* saying that the best way to balance your hormones is to eat lots of fatty foods; just the opposite, in fact.

*The right treat can make you feel extra good*
*and help balance your hormones at the same time.*

Foods that are high in saturated fats and trans fats are clearly unhealthy choices. To make matters worse, they can throw other hormones—in particular, insulin—out of balance. It is important to know, however, that on those occasions when you choose a special treat, you might find that pudding, ice cream, chocolate, and the like can boost your levels of oxytocin and help balance your adrenaline levels, too.

Few scientists understand the connection, but you can get a similar oxytocin boost from the capsaicin in chile pepper. You might want to eat them in moderation, however, to prevent a rebound of adrenaline. Want a quick and simple way of boosting oxytocin? Scientists have discovered that sensible supplementation with vitamin C can do the trick, as well.

*Vitamin C can increase your sex drive?*
*Now, that's interesting!*

# VITAMIN C: IT MAY IMPROVE YOUR SEX DRIVE!

In a groundbreaking study, Stuart Brody, PhD, of the Institute for Medical Psychology and Behavioral Neurobiology, discovered that high-dose supplements of vitamin C increased oxytocin release, improved mood, and boosted women's interest in sexual intercourse—all at the same time!

We would caution you against going out and consuming high doses of vitamin C in the hopes of experiencing any of the benefits above (or all of them). The appropriateness and safety of high doses have *not* been established.

Currently, we are researching the hypotheses that *recommended* levels of vitamin C supplementation, along with foods rich in vitamin C (such as citrus fruits), may help raise oxytocin levels in the Quicky Stress-Eater. The research looks promising, but it's too early to come to any definitive conclusions at this time.

For now, your path is clear: Begin the Stress-Eating Cure Program (Chapters 21 through 29). Within the guidelines of the program—whenever you can and as often as possible—indulge yourself in the hormone-balancing goodness of pure pleasure.

# 40

# The Delayed
# Stress-Eater's Cure

## YOUR PERSONALIZED PLAN

### Getting Started

The recommendations you find within this chapter have been individualized specifically for the Delayed Stress-Eater. To turn the Stress-Eating Cure Program into your personalized Stress-Eating Cure, simply apply these recommendations to the Stress-Eating Cure Program (Chapters 21 through 29).

In the hormonally *balanced* body, three words describe the natural reaction of Delayed Stress-Eating: *appropriate*, *useful*, and *time-limited*.

Delayed Stress-Eating is an *appropriate* response to a stressful situation. When faced with a threat, it makes perfect sense that the body would channel its energy away from the digestive processes and make that same blood and energy available to the muscles and nervous system, which are more likely to be called into action. After all, it is unlikely that, when faced with a real life-or-death threat, any of us would think it wise to stop for a snack.

Delayed Stress-Eating is *useful* in replenishing the energy that might have been used in a fight-or-flight experience. If you have been running for your life or fighting for it, after the danger has passed, it's a very good idea to chow down all the food that might be available in order to refill the quick energy you might soon need again.

Delayed Stress-Eating is *time-limited,* and it is this characteristic more than any other that sets it apart from Stress-Eating Patterns that can lead to self-perpetuating Stress-Eating Cycles.

Within a short time after a stressful experience is over, cortisol levels begin to normalize. Cortisol's hormonal partners—ghrelin, leptin, insulin, serotonin, and others—return to ideal levels as well. Those hormones that may still remain somewhat high or low are usually brought back into balance by the act of eating itself.

*Where there is a natural return to balance,*
*there is no need for any intervention.*

In a state of hormonal balance, should stress continue for a prolonged period or if it is replaced by new stressors, cortisol levels may rise, but not excessively. They are likely to stay within a high-normal range for a limited time depending on an individual's genetic makeup and the intensity of the stress. As soon as the Delayed Stress-Eater becomes accustomed to the demanding situation(s), however, cortisol levels will usually return to normal.

As hormones go, so goes the eating. Without any intervention, normal eating patterns will usually return naturally. For the body in hormonal balance, the Delayed Stress-Eater has no need for a personalized plan.

## WHEN ALL DOES *NOT* GO AS IT SHOULD

On the other hand, when normal, prestress eating patterns do *not* return naturally, a significant hormonal imbalance is likely to be present.

New eating patterns not marked by a healthy ebb-and-flow of hunger followed after eating, or by a feeling of satisfaction and the disappearance of the desire to eat, may be signs of a hormonal imbalance. Fortunately, the Stress-Eating Cure Program can help reset the hormonal balance to prestress levels.

Here's how to get started: Begin the basic Stress-Eating Cure Program by reading Chapters 21 through 29, then choose either the Step-by-Step Plan or the Quick-Start Plan and get started.

With your hormonal balance back to prestress levels, when stress reemerges, the body should be far more able to put eating on hold. With hormones in balance, eating is likely to remain on hold until the challenge of the moment has passed.

This hormonal give-and-take is the ideal, part of the natural order of the human body, and the goal of the Stress-Eating Cure Program. As you move into longer and longer periods that are free from stress-hunger and cravings, as the excess weight drops off almost without effort, you will be able to face with a sense of confidence the stresses that life may bring.

Certainly, your genetics and your hormones can have great power over you. Ultimately, however, knowing how to bring them back into balance with the program that follows, you have the final say!

# PART
# VI

# 41

# Stress-Eating Busters

Stress-Eating Busters are tips, strategies, actions, and activities that:

Balance your body

Clear your mind

Motivate your spirit

Stop the stress that can drive you to stress-eat

The Stress-Eating Busters you find in this chapter have been tried, tested, and proven. Some can change your body chemistry in only a moment; some can give you the boost you need to deal with impossible situations; most will become your best friends.

These are the tools you need to get you where you want to go. Some of the Stress-Eating Busters that you discover in this chapter may seem odd, while some may seem too easy, and others may seem too challenging.

We strongly urge you to try as many as you can, one at a time. They may surprise you—and, more than likely, you'll surprise yourself.

## COUNTERING COMFORT FOOD ACT-ALIKES: SABOTEURS TO SUCCESS

### Sugar Substitutes

You might be surprised to find that every time you popped some sugar-free chewing gum or an artificially sweetened mint into your mouth, you were "eating" a Comfort Food. The same goes with juice drinks, power drinks, flavored water, and sodas that contain sugar substitutes—*any* sugar substitute.

*If it contains a sugar substitute, it can set you up to stress-eat.*

This is not to say that *all* Comfort Foods are sweet. Some may not have the slightest trace of sweetness, yet if eaten frequently, they can set off hormonal imbalances that lead to stress-eating.

On the other hand, if a food or beverage *does* taste sweet, even though its sweetness does not come from sugar, most definitely consider it a Comfort Food. And be aware that if consumed throughout the day, it can send your stress-hunger and cravings soaring.

The idea that sugar substitutes can sabotage your weight-loss success might seem odd to some people. But not when you look at the scientific research rather than the advertising.

*Suppose scientists discovered that diet soda
could make you fat and sick. Wouldn't you expect to
hear it on the evening news?*

In 2007, a team of researchers from Harvard University, Brigham and Women's Hospital, Boston University School of Medicine, Tufts University, and other prestigious institutions reported on the incidence of metabolic syndrome among soda drinkers and non–soda drinkers. Metabolic syndrome (also known as Syndrome X) is a hormonal imbalance that is marked by obesity, excess fat around the waist, diabetes, high blood pressure, cardiovascular disease, and other medical conditions. Among soda drinkers, the findings were astounding: The likelihood of developing metabolic syndrome was far higher in those who consumed one or more diet sodas a day than in those who consumed equal quantities of sugar-laden sodas; in fact, the risk was a full 50 to 60 percent higher in the diet soda drinkers!

In 2009, scientists presenting at the annual meeting of the Endocrine Society reported even more remarkable findings. Their study compared two groups that took in the same number of calories and equivalent amounts of fat and carbohydrates. Though food intake was the same, the group that consumed sugar substitutes was significantly fatter and had significantly higher glucose (blood sugar) levels than the group that didn't consume sugar substitutes.

Scientists from the University of Minnesota School of Public Health in Minneapolis and the University of North Carolina, Department of Nutrition in Chapel Hill confirmed the diet soda connection to hormonal imbalances, obesity, and metabolic syndrome in their 2008 study published in the esteemed medical journal *Circulation*. The researchers noted, "Diet soda also was positively associated with incident metabolic syndrome, with those in the highest tertile of intake at 34 percent greater risk."

*High blood pressure, blood sugar problems,*
*even the fat around your middle*
*might all be related to your diet drinks!*

These researchers went on to report that their findings "were consistent with recent data from the Framingham Heart Study, which found a 56 percent increased risk of metabolic syndrome among those consuming one serving of diet soda a day."

"Furthermore," they added, "in a recent cross-sectional study, diabetics who consumed diet soda had poorer glucose control than those who consumed none."

The reason for the obesity and hormonal imbalance connection to diet soda (and sugar substitutes in general) is pretty apparent. The human body was never built to handle sweeteners that are 300 times as sweet as sugar. Sugar substitutes shock the system, especially in those who are genetically sensitive to their hormonal impact. The body reacts as it would to any stress, pulling the stress-eater into a powerful cycle of stress-hunger, cravings, stress-eating, and enhanced weight gain.

It is unfortunate that scientific findings of such importance as these, studies that link the intake of just one diet soda a day to a far greater risk for the hormonal imbalances that are associated with obesity and a cluster of life-endangering disorders are never revealed to the public. In general, this groundbreaking research gets virtually no air time on the very TV news shows that air diet soda commercials.

You, however, now know the truth. If you'd like to do something about it but don't know if you can, we might just have the solution in the following Stress-Eating Buster.

### Diet Soda Liberation (without the Stress)

Let's imagine that giving up sugar substitutes is something you'd like to try but that you are unsure if you can do it—or how to go about it. Here's a suggestion that we have found works well.

Instead of imposing stress-filled demands on yourself to give up your diet drinks, we suggest you try the following for a few days: Whenever you think of having a diet soda or a sugar-free dessert, gum, or mint (one that has been sweetened with sugar substitutes), *ask* yourself if you could possibly do without it.

Don't push yourself. Don't *demand* that you give up a diet soda when you *really* want it. On the other hand, if you're drinking a diet soda out of habit or because it happens to be handy, consider having a seltzer, a cold glass of water, or iced tea (with no sweetener of any kind) instead.

Make it a matter of preference. If you really want a diet soda, have it. If you could live without it, make a choice to pass it up.

We have found that with this approach, each successive day will bring fewer and fewer choices that involve drinks with sugar substitutes.

Always "ask" yourself to forgo the sugar substitute, but do not demand compliance. In some cases, commanding yourself to give up diet soda may be more stressful than the diet soda itself. Clearly, stress rebound is not the goal.

On the other hand, a simple request to yourself to cut down, cut back, and then let go of sugar substitutes when possible will often go a great deal further than you might imagine.

In a few days, as you are able to choose more and more often to pass on the diet soda, as your hormone levels regain their natural balance, your newly emerging feelings of freedom will help ensure your continuing success. What might have been a challenge in the past can easily become a part of your new way of eating and living.

As always, consult with your physician before making major changes in your eating program—including the cessation of sugar substitutes.

# Glutamates

Some stress-eaters think that they can pretty much avoid MSG (monosodium glutamate) in their food by requesting that their meals at restaurants contain no MSG and by checking labels on their foods. If you consider that this is a reasonable way to avoid the hunger-producing and weight-gaining power of MSG, consider this:

> Unless you have been eating 100 percent natural foods that are grown and milled and prepared by you alone, and only if you never eat at a restaurant, put a mint or stick of gum in your mouth, or use toothpaste or mouthwash can you be reasonably certain of not falling under the influence of MSG or some other glutamate.

There's no escaping it. It's a part of life in this culture.

There is help and hope, however. If you know how to spot MSG in your food, how to avoid it when you can, how to recognize its effects on your stress-eating and your weight, and what to do to counter its impact, you stand a good chance at keeping your MSG intake as minimal as possible.

### So, What's So Bad about MSG?

MSG, as well as other glutamates, can appear in food naturally, but food manufacturers now routinely add glutamates to enhance the flavors of foods. Some food manufacturers (that term seems to say it all) apparently have applied for and been granted EPA approval to spray crops with a mixture that is 29.2 percent pharmaceutical-grade glutamic acid (MSG). In this way, you can be sold a fresh or prepared product that bears a no-MSG-added label but which in fact could contain several times the amount of MSG than that which might otherwise be added to your food.

Why the push by food manufacturers to include MSG in your food? The answer is simple and, as often is the case, comes down to profits. MSG and its cousin glutamates cause hormonal responses that compel people to develop a strong preference for a food and to consume a great deal of it.

Although it is labeled as a taste-enhancer, MSG does far more than make food taste good. It makes you want to eat the food even if you don't particularly like it. So if you've ever been drawn to a food, if you've ever kept eating a certain food even though you weren't really enjoying it that much, chances are it contained a good portion of MSG or some other glutamate.

Without knowing it, you may be selecting brands that contain higher levels of added glutamates, not because these foods taste better or because they satisfy you more fully, but rather because the glutamates they contain are throwing your hormones out of balance and pulling you into a Stress-Eating Cycle that includes that particular food.

Food manufacturers have long known that we have glutamate receptors in our taste buds. These receptors drive us to seek out and consume foods that contain glutamates even when we cannot actually taste the glutamates.

Glutamates seem to enhance other tastes as well as the sensation of eating—but at a price.

*When scientists want obese lab animals for experiments, they can get rats that were made fat by feeding them MSG.*

Glutamates are categorized as excitotoxins, that is, they cause injury or death by stimulation. When added to food, glutamates can have powerful consequences. They break down muscle fiber and cause brain damage in laboratory animals.

In humans and laboratory animals, the result is the same: altered levels of leptin, insulin, and ghrelin, three of the hormones that drive you to eat, tell you when to stop (or fail to tell you to stop), and tell your body whether to store the food energy you take in or to burn it.

Did you know that scientists who want obese lab animals for experimentation call the supply house and ask for MSG-fattened rats? The rats become obese simply by eating feed to which monosodium glutamate has been added!

Though they may hit opposition from vested interests, scientists, such as those at the Department of Nutrition at the University of North Carolina at Chapel Hill, confirmed these findings in 2009 and reported, "This research provides data that MSG intake may be associated with increased risk of overweight independent of physical activity and total energy intake in humans."

These researchers, and many others, are beginning to understand that, regardless of the type and amount of food that is eaten or the activity in which they participate, some people can get fat from eating foods containing MSG.

The problem is, you might be eating foods saturated with MSG without ever knowing it. Food that you have been buying in the same cans and packages, with labels that do not appear to have changed, may contain one or more newly added glutamates.

*When they took the oil out of canned tuna,*
*they put the MSG in.*

One of the most obvious examples is the canned fish industry. Several years ago, when tuna manufacturers felt the pressure to replace oil-packed tuna with a water-packed variety, they faced a major dilemma.

While consumers clearly preferred the water-pack for health reasons, this variety was decidedly less tasty than its oil-based predecessor. Food manufacturers solved their problem by adding free glutamates (chemicals that are very similar in structure to monosodium glutamate), which not only enhanced the flavor of the water-packed tuna but also did not appear to the consumer to be as "unhealthy" as oil.

Added under one of a dozen names, one or more glutamates began appearing in the ingredient labels of virtually every major brand of canned tuna, even though the front of the can still sported the familiar "tuna in spring water" label. Unsuspecting consumers never knew—nor do most realize to this day—that while they were being so "good" on their weight-reduction diets, they were actually ingesting chemicals that could be interfering with their best efforts to control their eating and promote their weight loss.

While it is relatively easy to avoid many food additives by reading the ingredient label, in the United States, it is much more difficult to detect the addition of glutamates, which may be included under so many names that to really know what you're eating, you have to compare the nutritional label with the long list on page 234.

To make matters even more difficult for the unsuspecting consumer, many of the alternate names used for glutamates may appear very benign, even healthy, including "broth" and "natural flavors."

You may have been eating these foods, assuming that something labeled "natural flavors" should not cause concern, and never have imagined that so healthy-sounding an ingredient might come back to haunt you in the form of stress-hunger, cravings, and weight gain.

After all, you might reason, if it's natural, what can be bad about it? Our response to this question is not meant to be harsh but rather to bring home a point: If you think natural is good, consider the fact that cyanide, arsenic, and dirt are also natural, but no one would want them added to their food.

The problem is that the deceptively innocent image of anything called "natural flavors" or "broth" is difficult to counter. Only a few of the low-salt, low-calorie varieties of canned tuna contain no glutamates. You can spot the glutamate-free brands because the ingredient list on the label (not the starburst on the front of the can) reads: tuna, water (and nothing else).

> *Look at a can of tuna. If the ingredient list includes*
> *broth or hydrolyzed protein, you could end up*
> *stress-eating before you've finished the meal.*

While some manufacturers may not lie, they don't always tell the entire truth. When we called the top two manufacturers of canned tuna fish, we were told that no monosodium glutamate had been added. When we asked specifically if free glutamates were added, both companies confirmed our suspicion.

Though each manufacturer knew that, for our purposes, there was almost no difference between free glutamates and monosodium glutamate, both companies refused to admit the presence of this additive until they were forced to do so.

Fortunately, we have found that tuna and other canned fish packed in olive oil usually does not contain glutamates. Perhaps that's because it tastes good enough without a chemical sledgehammer to back it up.

While some may claim that there is nothing wrong with glutamates, we say if you are trying to balance your hormones, stop stress-eating, and lose weight, stay away from MSG and all other added glutamates. These chemicals may alter your hormones of metabolism, slow down your weight loss, and drive you solidly into a Stress-Eating Cycle—all without you ever knowing why.

If you are having repeated problems getting on or staying on the Stress-Eating Cure Program, if stress-eating just seems to take over at times, if your weight loss is slow or marked by plateaus, carefully check the ingredient labels on the foods you've been eating.

Almost invariably you'll discover the source of your problem in the many glutamates you had been consuming under a host of names. When these foods are substituted with brands that do not contain glutamates or with fresh foods, a renewed sense of calm and control can return in a matter of only a few days.

*Seventy-five percent of all restaurant meals contain added glutamates. To minimize the MSG, choose unprocessed foods such as chicken or steak without gravies or sauces.*

Added glutamates appear to be more of a problem for stress-eaters than naturally occurring glutamates. Unfortunately, if you eat out, you probably can't avoid glutamates altogether. It is estimated that three-quarters or more of all the food you eat in restaurants contains added glutamates. This explains why, in part, some of us tend to put on a pound or two (or more) after eating out.

You are forced to put up with glutamates in order to live a normal life, but when you have a choice, when you buy food in grocery stores, try the following Stress-Eating Buster.

### Glutamates: Avoid and Conquer

It's important to read the label and, whenever possible, avoid food with added glutamates. Always look at that part of the label that has the list of ingredients—not the splash or banner label on the front or side that tells you what the food manufacturer wants you to think is true.

233

Food manufacturers add glutamates by including any of the following ingredients:

| | |
|---|---|
| Anything enzyme-modified | Hydrolyzed vegetable protein |
| Anything fermented | Malt extract |
| Anything protein-fortified | Maltodextrin |
| Anything ultra-pasteurized | Natural flavors or flavoring |
| Autolyzed yeast | Pectin |
| Barley malt | Plant protein extract |
| Bouillon | Potassium glutamate |
| Broth | Sodium caseinate |
| Calcium caseinate | Soy protein |
| Carrageenan | Soy sauce |
| Flavoring | Stock |
| Gelatin | Textured protein |
| Hydrolyzed oat flour | Whey protein |
| Hydrolyzed plant protein | Yeast extract |
| Hydrolyzed soy protein | Yeast food |

As the world progresses, it doesn't make sense to live in fear of added glutamates. There is virtually no way to avoid them entirely. In order to keep your hormones on an even keel, your stress-hunger and cravings down, and your weight dropping, however, it would be wise to avoid glutamates *when you can.*

When they cannot be avoided, it makes sense to take in a good portion of water or sparkling water at the same time in hopes of flushing the system and to avoid other food-related stressors (such as caffeine, sugar, sugar substitutes, and saturated or trans fats) at the same meal.

We have found that a nap after exposure to MSG makes you feel better and that the meal that follows is best when it contains Balancing Proteins and Balancing Vegetables and/or Salad only.

Remember, if something you eat gives you a "hit," even though you know it's not the finest in culinary cuisine, you are probably feeling the effects of the added glutamates. Avoid it if you can. Counter it if you must.

Trust what your body is trying to tell you and, most important, learn from each experience.

*No time to exercise? No real desire to, either?*
*No problem! Try these!*

# MORE STRESS-EATING BUSTERS: ACTIVITIES THAT ENHANCE

Hormone-Balancing Activities are actions you can take to get the most out of your Stress-Eating Cure Program. With very little time but a bit of ingenuity, you can ensure that you will remain stress-eating free and increase your weight loss at the same time.

## Traditional Activities

Traditional activities and exercises, such as walking, jogging, weight training, swimming, dancing, stretching, and biking (stationary or street), are excellent activities that can help keep your hormones right on target.

You need not burn calories by the hundreds to get the desired effect. In fact, overdoing your workouts could cause more stress and hormonal rebound than no exercise at all.

We have found that a short workout every day rather than a greater workout every 2 days seems to work best for the stress-eater.

We don't think it's possible to offer recommendations regarding the ideal duration of activity or exercise for you. Each person reading this page has different activity needs, different goals, and, most important, a body that is like no one else's.

Certainly, check with your physician and, as advisable with monitoring, begin to increase the duration and intensity of your activity, preferably every day (with time out for weekends, perhaps!).

Remember, the goal is not to qualify for the Olympics. Just increase your activity level in order to get your body moving and your hormones humming.

# Nontraditional Activities

### Coffee Break Calisthenics

Use your coffee break to do a few situps, jumping jacks, pushups, or other muscle-toning exercises.

In the 15 minutes you would usually use to down a doughnut and set off your cravings, you can build muscle, improve your cardiovascular system, and give your stress-eating resistance a real shot in the arm.

### Elevator Bends and Stretches

If you take the elevator regularly, you can fit a simple Stress-Eating Buster into your day, every day.

While waiting for the elevator or traveling in it, complete one stretching exercise that can be performed standing up.

Too many people around? No problem. Make it a game of sleuth and opportunity. Find yourself a place in the back of the crowd where no one can see you, and stretch away.

The excitement of getting away with your secret pursuit can add spice to the activity.

If you want more privacy, wait for the next elevator or take an elevator in the wrong direction. Go a bit farther than the other passenger and you've just grabbed yourself a few extra minutes.

We won't advise you to stop the elevator at an empty floor for a few stolen moments, but we will say that if you do, we won't tell.

If you take the elevator several times a day, these few minutes of fun and stretching each time can really add up.

### Wet and Wild Shower Workouts

Your wake-up shower doesn't have to be dull. Mornings are the best time to help balance your hormones (as your Big Balanced Breakfast can attest).

Don't just lean on the shower wall and dream of going back to bed. Don't just stand under the running water and list all of the challenges that you are about to face in the day ahead.

Twist and stretch while you soap yourself up. After a warmup of stretching, gently, and as appropriate, move into some deep knee bends while you rinse off. Let the warm water help you flex and bring some action into your shower stall.

Take care that you don't slip, of course, or overdo your activity so early in the day. With that said, however, you can have fun in the shower and do your hormones a favor as well.

### Morning Mattress Isometrics

Isometrics are fundamental to yoga and Chinese martial arts. They were big in the sixties and they're coming back into fashion. Check them out, and if they're right for you, give them a new twist: Take them to the mattress!

While some isometric exercises must be done in standing, stooping, or bending positions, others can be done in a prone position.

Get up 5 or 10 minutes early, and as you're lying in bed watching TV or listening to the radio, bring on the isometrics. Start with some stretches to warm up. Take care to not overdo, and choose those activities that are appropriate to you and your limitations.

You'll enjoy a few extra minutes to yourself in the morning, and when you hit the ground, you'll be ready to take on the day.

# EVEN MORE STRESS-EATING BUSTERS: ADVENTURES THAT AUGMENT

Hormone-balancing adventures are experiences that bring additional balance and stress-resilience to your body. Some are traditional, thousands of years old. Some are contemporary, clearly unusual, meant to balance . . . always, and to intrigue and titillate as well.

## Traditional Activities

Traditional hormone-balancing activities include power naps, guided imagery, deep-breathing techniques, massage, increased sleep time, journal-keeping, and standard relaxation techniques, among others.

No single activity is right for all stress-eaters. You are likely to find that some hold personal appeal for you while others are clearly less desirable.

If any traditional experience is of interest, make time to pursue it. Though it might be impossible to fit in an extra hour or two of sleep each night, you may discover that a 10-minute power nap or a regular massage can do you a great deal of good.

On the other hand, some nontraditional activities might hold far more interest.

# Nontraditional Activities

### Instant Media Gratification

The pleasure you get from a TV show or movie can reach deep and de-stress you from the inside out. The only problem is that few people, especially stress-eaters, take time to take advantage of this instant feel-good remedy.

If at all possible, invest in a personal, portable DVD player. If you have not done so already, begin to assemble your very own library of DVDs or, as an alternative, if finances allow, join a DVD rental club.

Then, most importantly, make time to take advantage of the enjoyment that you have coming. Hang on some earphones and make your favorite TV show a part of your lunch break. If you have an MP3 player, listen to some music or an audio book. Take some time in the evening just for yourself. Put everyone else on hold and, while your hormones rebalance, have a real good time.

> Music hath charms to soothe the savage breast,
> To soften rocks, or bend a knotted oak.
> *William Congreve* (1670–1729)

### The Bathroom Fix

In some ways, this adventure is similar to Instant Media Gratification, but this adventure costs less, is available at a moment's notice, and takes only 5 minutes.

It takes advantage of those songs that, when you hear the first strains of the music, make you sigh and relax into the pleasure of hearing them. Apparently, they can do a great deal more than just make you feel good; they can help get you and keep you slim.

The right song can do wonders to bring your hormones back in line. So, plan for pleasure. Load up your MP3 player with your favorite songs (then remember to take it with you to work).

When things get strained at work, head for the bathroom (with your MP3 player hidden from view). There, in the privacy of your stall, hook on your earphones and relax into the music that helps and heals.

It's easy to keep track of the time. Play a couple of your favorites or the same tune two or three times.

When you return to the tasks at hand with your hormones back in balance, your body will be far more able to handle the stress. Your stress-hunger, cravings, and drive to stress-eat will have been eliminated at the source. And no one will ever suspect the secret to your serenity.

Next time you feel like reaching for a doughnut, reach for your MP3 player instead and head for a few minutes of pure me-time!

### Hot Creature Comforts

It's simple physics: Cold contracts, heat relaxes. What heat does to all else in the world, it does to you. And the relaxation that heat brings translates into better hormonal balance.

A hot shower is a great way to start the day. It's especially helpful given that morning is the time of your greatest hormonal imbalance. But what about the rest of the day?

You can't very well go running off to the shower every time you hit a stressful situation. Or can you?

We have found that a 2-minute "mini-shower" of warm water applied directly to the inside of your wrists can do wonders to relax you, relieve pressure, and return your hormones to their rightful balance.

So take full use of your bathroom break (again!). Let the warm water wash away the stresses of the day, your urge to stress-eat, and the pounds that can result, all at the same time.

Evening brings opportunity for a special variation on this Stress-Eating Buster. The bath: hot, luxurious, relaxing, rejuvenating, and a hormonal blessing.

The Romans had it right. They built huge bathhouses complete with plumbing, hot water, and room heating. The main purpose of these palaces of pleasure was far more than the attainment of cleanliness. The enjoyment of the bath was an integral part of the culture, payback for a hard day at work, rejuvenation of the mind, body, and spirit. In other words, a good destressing!

The Roman philosopher Cicero wrote, "The gong that announced the opening of the public baths each day was a sweeter sound than the voices of the philosophers in their school." Why should you not experience the same pleasure they knew 2,000 years ago?

We have made a hot bath part of our everyday life. Each night, when our research and writing responsibilities are completed, we slip into our double bathtub and allow the warm water to heal us and wash away the tensions of the day.

At the foot of the bath, we have arranged a VHS player, a DVD player, and a flat-screen TV (at a safe distance). There we sit and soak, watch and relax, and simply allow in the pleasure the warm water brings. Like the hot springs of years gone by, our baths allow us to emerge restored and stress-free.

When finances were tight, we timed our baths to coincide with our favorite evening TV shows, set the television on the toilet seat, and, facing each other, squeezed into our single-person claw-foot bathtub. Clearly, where there is a will for pleasure, there is a way!

## Sex and Masturbation

This Stress-Eating Buster comes with quite a bit of encouragement but no instructions!

Sex and masturbation can be great tension-relievers and a perfect way to restore your hormonal balance. 'Nuff said.

*Too often, today's slip becomes*
*tomorrow's accepted way of eating.*

# STRESS-EATING FIRST AID: WHAT TO DO IF YOU SLIP

Many people find the Stress-Eating Cure Program so easy that they don't seem overly concerned with the possibility of a slip; that is, eating outside of the program guidelines. We have a somewhat different attitude.

We believe that it is very important to stay vigilant. If you slip today, if you eat Comfort Foods in meals or snacks that are meant to include Balancing Foods only, you could be setting yourself up to slip back into a Stress-Eating Cycle.

Take every slip seriously. At the same time, don't blame yourself for it. Learn from it!

When you realize that you have slipped, stop what you're doing and take a good look at what you were feeling and needing as well as what you might have been feeling stressed by. Carefully scrutinize the foods you had been eating; in many cases, you will find that although you thought they were Balancing Foods, they contained Comfort Food Act-Alikes such as glutamates or sugar substitutes.

Consider how tired you might have been and what other stresses you were facing and then—now, here's the most important part—do something to prevent the slip from happening again.

Quite honestly, it's not enough to just say that you were tired and that's why you grabbed a doughnut and downed it before you knew what was happening. What happens the next time you're tired?

Some of us have quite ingenious minds. Knowing that Comfort Foods may lie as a reward at the end of a sleep-deprived night, we might unconsciously repeat the behavior in order to have an excuse to eat whatever we like.

Even those who are not quite that ingenious in their premeditation can find they fall into a pattern of "becauses." A "because" is a logical-*sounding* reason that serves as a justification for going off your program. "I ate that *because* I was tired," you might say. Or "*because* I had a fight with my husband" or "*because* I was sick of the same food every day."

The problem with "becauses" is that they don't lead to a solution.

They accomplish their purpose: to make you feel that your slip was understandable and, at the same time, imply that this was an unusual circumstance, one that is not likely to recur.

The truth is, there is likely to never be a day when you aren't tired or at odds with a mate or family member or when you aren't seeking some new and exciting foods. Or a hundred other reasons that, on a moment's notice, can be served up as a handy "because."

Rather than asking yourself *why* you went off your program, we strongly suggest you ask yourself what could have been done to *prevent* yourself from slipping.

"I need to get more sleep" will get you halfway to preventing future slips. The second half comes from immediately following the analysis with a plan of action. "I will make certain that, no matter what, I'm in bed by 11:00 p.m."

If you follow through on your plan to get more sleep, for example, you will have eliminated one "because" from the list. One by one, as your "becauses" fall away, your program will become more consistent and the benefits far greater.

If, on the other hand, you do not follow through on the change you plan, you will be able to see, at an instant, that the reason was not just that you were tired but that you didn't use enough healthy selfishness to put your own needs first.

### After the slip, how do I get back on track?

One of the most frequently asked questions we encounter is how to get back into the program after a slip. The answer depends on the duration of the slip and how intense it was. Most important, it depends on whether or not your stress-hunger, cravings, and stress-eating have returned.

If your breach on the program was a single incident and if you are not experiencing ongoing impulses to stress-eat, just pick yourself up, dust yourself off, figure out what went wrong, correct it, and go back to the program where you left it.

On the other hand, if your slip ended up going on for more than a day or you are experiencing strong impulses to stress-eat or are caught in a Stress-Eating Cycle, you might need to go back to Step #1 and start from the beginning.

*Don't start over, start smarter.*

If you need to start the program fresh, from Step #1, you have two choices. If you know the program well and you can follow the guidelines consistently, you need not stay at any step for more than 1 day. If, however, you have not been consistent with any step, stay there until you get it right for 2 full days. Don't linger more than a short time, but do stay an extra day or two if necessary to get it right.

Of greatest importance, however, is to be certain that *before* you start the program again, you do all that can be done to eliminate the stress that first set off your slip.

If you followed the Quick-Start Plan to enter the program and this is your second or third slip (or more), we strongly recommend that you move into the Step-by-Step Plan. It may seem as if you are moving more slowly, but, in the end, it may well get you to your goal more quickly. Better yet, it may help to keep you there for good.

# 42

# Food Lists You'll Need to Succeed

Balancing Foods are listed on the following four pages in two sections: Balancing Proteins and Balancing Vegetables and Salad.

## BALANCING PROTEINS LIST

All choices should comply with your physician's recommendations regarding dietary fat, nitrates, and other relevant health concerns.

### Meats

All meats, including the leanest portions possible of:

| | |
|---|---|
| Bacon, Canadian only | Lunch meats[1] |
| Beef | Pork |
| Ham | Rabbit |
| Hamburger | Sausages[1] |
| Hot dogs[1] | Veal |
| Lamb | Venison |

### Fowl

All varieties, light or dark meat, with or without skin, including:

| | |
|---|---|
| Capon | Duck |
| Chicken[2] | Goose |
| Cornish hen | Pheasant |

---

[1] Containing no added sugars, fillers, added saturated fats, or trans fats
[2] Regular or luncheon meat

## Fowl, continued

Quail

Squab

Turkey[2]

## Fish and Shellfish[3]

All varieties including:

| | |
|---|---|
| Bass | Oysters |
| Bluefish | Perch |
| Calamari | Salmon |
| Clams | Sardines |
| Cod | Scallops |
| Crabmeat | Scrod |
| Flounder | Shrimp |
| Haddock | Smelt |
| Halibut | Sole |
| Herring | Sturgeon |
| Lobster | Swordfish |
| Monk | Trout |
| Mussels | Tuna |

## Nuts and Seeds

All varieties as well as nut butters[1] made from:

| | |
|---|---|
| Almonds | Pine nuts |
| Butternuts | Pistachios |
| Cashews | Pumpkin seeds |
| Chestnuts | Sesame seeds |
| Hazelnuts | Squash seeds |
| Macadamias | Sunflower seeds |
| Peanuts | Walnuts |
| Pecans | |

---

[3] Natural shellfish only (not artificial substitutes)

# BALANCING PROTEINS LIST (CONTINUED)

## Dairy and Non-Meat Alternatives[4]

Regular or low-fat varieties of:

Eggs, egg whites, or
egg substitutes

Milk (fat-free, 1%, 2%, whole,
cream, or half-and-half)

Sour cream

Tofu (soybean curd)

Cheese (all varieties, low-fat
or regular), including:

American

Blue

Brick

Brie

Camembert

Caraway

Cheddar

Cottage cheese
(regular or creamed)

Cream cheese

Edam

Feta

Goat cheese

Gouda

Gruyère

Monterey Jack

Mozzarella

Muenster

Neufchâtel

Parmesan

Provolone

Ricotta

Swiss

## Unsaturated Fats and Oils[5]

Olive oil[6]

Canola oil

Corn oil

Cottonseed oil

Flaxseed oil

Omega-3 oils

Omega-6 oils

Peanut oil

Safflower oil

Sesame oil

Soybean oil

Sunflower oil

---

[4] Containing no added sugars, fillers, added saturated fats, or trans fats
[5] Not all oils are suitable for cooking.
[6] Olive oil is a highly preferred, multiuse monounsaturated oil.

# BALANCING VEGETABLES AND SALAD LIST

*Important note:* If a vegetable or salad ingredient is not listed below, do *not* consider it to be a Balancing Food.

The following vegetables may be served raw or cooked:

| | |
|---|---|
| Alfalfa sprouts | Greens (all) |
| Arugula | Kale |
| Asparagus | Kohlrabi |
| Bamboo shoots | Lettuce (all) |
| Bean sprouts | Mushroom |
| Bok choy | Okra |
| Broccoli | Parsley |
| Brussels sprouts | Peppers, green |
| Cabbage (red and green) | Radishes |
| Cauliflower | Scallions |
| Celery | Snap beans |
| Cucumbers | Sorrel |
| Daikon | Sour grass |
| Endive | Spinach |
| Green beans | Wax beans |

## Condiments in a Class of Their Own

Small amounts of the following ingredients, used in cooking, can be included in Balancing Food dishes.

| | |
|---|---|
| Cornstarch | Marsala wine |
| Cream of tartar | Soy sauce |
| Hot-pepper sauce | Teriyaki |
| Lemon juice | Wine |

# COMFORT FOODS LIST

This list contains a sampling of the many Comfort Foods you can enjoy on this program. It is impossible to list all possible Comfort Foods in a list of reasonable length. Assume that any foods not listed in the Balancing Foods lists are Comfort Foods.

Be sure to include Comfort Foods (along with Balancing Foods) in your Big Balanced Breakfasts or in your Alternative Meals. All choices should comply with your physician's recommendations regarding dietary fat, sugars, and other relevant health concerns.

## Breads, Grains, Cereals, and Legumes

Bagels

Beans (see Legumes)

Biscuits

Breading

Breads

Breakfast bars

Cereals (hot or cold)

Cornmeal

Couscous

Crackers

Croissants

English muffins

Flatbreads

French toast

Granola

Grits

Lentils

Legumes, all varieties other than green or wax beans, including baked beans, chickpeas, kidney, and lima

Matzo

Pancakes

Panini

Rolls

Stuffing

Tabbouleh

Tahini

Tempura coating

Waffles

Water chestnuts

# Fruits and Juices

All varieties, fresh, juiced, or dried, including:

| | |
|---|---|
| Apples and juice | Lemons |
| Apricots and juice | Limes |
| Bananas | Mangoes |
| Cantaloupe | Oranges |
| Carrot juice | Papayas |
| Cherries | Peaches |
| Cider | Pears |
| Coconut | Pineapples and juice |
| Dates | Plums |
| Figs | Prunes and juice |
| Grapefruit | Raisins |
| Grapes and juice | V-8 juices |
| Kiwifruit | |

# Dairy

Varieties *not* included in the Balancing Proteins list, including sugar-sweetened and sugar-free:

| | |
|---|---|
| Creamers (nondairy) | Ice milk |
| Food replacement drinks | Yogurt (flavored, fruited, or |
| Ice cream | frozen) |

# Protein Bars and Drinks

Sugar-sweetened, fruit juice added, or sugar-free[7] varieties:

| | |
|---|---|
| Food replacement bars | Protein drinks |
| Power bars | Soy protein powder and |
| Protein bars | drinks |

*(continued)*

---

[7] If you're wondering why sugar substitutes are included in the Comfort Foods list, see pages 225–28.

# COMFORT FOODS LIST (CONTINUED)

## Vegetables

All varieties *not* listed in the Balancing Foods list, including:

| | |
|---|---|
| Artichokes | Peas |
| Beets | Peppers (red) |
| Carrots | Potatoes |
| Corn | Squash |
| Leeks | Tomatoes |
| Onions | Zucchini |
| Pea pods | |

## Pasta, Rice, and Noodles

All varieties, including:

| | |
|---|---|
| Chinese noodles | Rigatoni |
| Egg noodles | Shells |
| Kasha | Spaghetti |
| Macaroni | Spinach noodles |
| Pasta | Tabbouleh |
| Rice | |

## Saturated Fats and Oils[8]

| | |
|---|---|
| Beef fat | Lard |
| Butter fat | Margarines with saturated fats |
| Chicken fat | Palm oil |
| Cocoa butter | Trans fats |
| Coconut oil | Vegetable shortening |
| Hydrogenated fats | |

---

[8] See Alcoholic Beverages and Saturated Fats on page 252.

## Snack Foods and Sweets

Sugar-sweetened or sugar-free[9] varieties:

| | |
|---|---|
| Cakes | Popcorn |
| Candy | Potato chips |
| Chocolate | Power bars |
| Cookies | Pretzels |
| Corn chips | Pudding |
| Crackers | Rice cakes |
| Danish | Snack bars |
| Doughnuts | Sugar |
| Gelatin desserts | Sugar substitutes |
| Honey | Toaster pastries |
| Meal replacement bars | Vegetable chips (containing |
| Mints | rice or corn) |
| Pastries | |

## Nonalcoholic Beverages and Extras

Sugar-sweetened or sugar-free[9] varieties:

| | |
|---|---|
| Barbecue sauce | Meal replacement drinks |
| Breath mints | Nonalcoholic beverages |
| Chewing gum | Sodas |
| Cough drops | Steak sauce |
| Ketchup | |

## Alcoholic Beverages[10]

All varieties of straight or mixed drinks, including:

| | |
|---|---|
| Apéritifs | Liquors |
| Beer | Wine |
| Champagne | |

---

[9] If you're wondering why sugar substitutes are included in the Comfort Foods list, see pages 225–28.

[10] See Alcoholic Beverages and Saturated Fats on page 252.

# ALCOHOLIC BEVERAGES AND SATURATED FATS

Alcohol and saturated fats should *not* be considered foods that give comfort, per se. They should be treated as Comfort Foods and are included in the Comfort Foods list because they can elicit similar hormonal imbalances as the sweet and starchy foods you will find here.

Alcoholic drinks should be consumed *only when appropriate and safe* and always as part of a well-balanced meal. When alcohol is not clearly appropriate as part of a Big Balanced Breakfast, it can be included in an Alternative Meal and consumed later in the day or evening.

Saturated fats such as trans fats, butter fat, beef fat, chicken fat, cocoa butter, coconut oil, lard, palm oil, hydrogenated fats, some margarines, and vegetable shortening should be avoided as much as possible and as per physician recommendations.

# Fat Facts at a Glance

Most fats and oils contain a mixture of two or more lipids. The fats and oils below are displayed according to their highest concentrations of a particular kind of fat.

This chart will help you spot those fats and oils that are least (and most) likely to throw your hormone levels out of kilter, increase your stress-hunger and cravings, or slow your weight loss.

| | High in Monounsaturated Fats | High in Polyunsaturated Fats | High in Saturated Fats | High in Trans Fatty Acids | |
|---|---|---|---|---|---|
| Best Choices: Least Likely to Lead to Hormonal Imbalances | Canola oil Olive oil (preferred) Peanut oil | Corn oil Cottonseed oil Omega-3 oils Omega-6 oils Safflower oil Sesame oil Soybean oil Sunflower oil | Beef fat Butter fat Chicken fat Cocoa butter Coconut oil Lard Milk fat Palm oil | Hydrogenated fats Some margarines Vegetable shortening | Undesirable Choices: Most Likely to Lead to Hormonal Imbalances |

Trans fats may be listed on ingredient labels as hydrogenated fats, partially hydrogenated fats, or trans *unsaturated* fats as well, even though processing has removed any of their former unsaturated-fat-related benefits. Don't be fooled by clever labeling.

In addition to their known potential to compromise heart health and increase the risk for cancer, trans fats and saturated fats have been shown to be detrimental to hormone balance. They can lead to stress-hunger, cravings, stress-eating, and weight-loss plateaus.

Whenever possible, unless otherwise advised by your physician, choose monounsaturated fats (or polyunsaturated fats) in place of saturated fats or trans fats.

# 43

# Recipes to Balance, Recipes to Comfort

The best way to guarantee that you will remain free of stress-eating for life is to make certain that you make everything you eat taste *really* good!

When it comes to Balancing Proteins and Balancing Vegetables and Salad, you may think you are just as happy having a plain piece of steak with some steamed vegetables or the same old salad day after day. Sooner or later, however, whether you are aware of it or not, you will get tired of it and you'll go looking for a little excitement.

Instead of realizing that you're getting tired of the same old uninteresting regime, you may tell yourself that your way of eating is "good enough" or, even worse, that it's "easy."

We have found that weight-loss success is not only about staying on track today; it's about putting enough energy into your program so that you find it *enjoyable* to stay on track tomorrow.

If you don't think that Balancing Proteins and Balancing Vegetables and Salad can be made interesting, you'd love dinner at our house. A typical meal for us starts off with a Shrimp Caliente appetizer, followed by a Chipotle Turkey Salad. The main course might include Luscious and Legal Lasagna and some Tangy Asian Pork Ribs (left over from yesterday). We always include a side plate of raw vegetables (to satisfy the need to crunch!) and our favorite Balancing Protein dip (such as Creamy Mustard Dipping Sauce). Green Beans Amandine round out the meal. You'll find all of these recipes in the pages that follow.

We've included some of our favorite Comfort Food recipes also: Unforgettable French Toast, Succulent Sweet-and-Sour Pork, Old-Fashioned Sour Cream Biscuits, Chocolate Silk, and more. If you're going to enjoy Comfort Foods once a day, they had better be worth the wait!

It's our hope that these recipes will provide a jumping-off place, a new start on your way to a life of balance—in all ways.

May you use them . . . to bring pleasure to yourself and to those you love.

May you change them . . . as you see fit.

May you add to them . . . with wonderful discoveries of your own.

May old favorites always be there when you need them and new surprises always bid you to explore.

Most of all, may you always give to yourself the energy, care, and consideration that you freely give to those you love.

# BALANCING FOOD RECIPES
## *BREAKFAST*
# Crustless Mushroom Quiche

*The creamy goodness of this quiche will help raise your oxytocin levels while reducing stress and bringing you pleasure. Save this rich dish for a special treat: a perfect appetizer at an Alternative Meal dinner or the Balancing Protein portion of a Big Balanced Breakfast.*

> 4 tablespoons olive oil
>
> 6 large mushroom caps, cleaned and sliced
>
> 1 cup light cream
>
> 1 cup grated cheese of choice
>
> 2 teaspoons dried basil
>
> ¾ teaspoon dried paprika
>
> 4 eggs (no low-fat substitutes)
>
> Salt and ground black pepper

Preheat the oven to 325°F.

Oil the bottom and sides of a 9" pie pan with 1 teaspoon of the olive oil. Set aside. Heat the remaining oil in a medium skillet over medium heat. Add the mushrooms and cook, stirring frequently, until tender. Drain and set aside.

Pour the cream into a medium saucepan and warm over medium-low heat until bubbles begin to form around the edges. Reduce the heat and stir in the cheese until melted. Stir in the basil and paprika.

Remove the saucepan from the heat and allow to cool for 5 minutes.

Add 1 egg at a time to the saucepan, mixing thoroughly until each is well distributed. Stir in the mushrooms and add salt and pepper to taste.

Pour the mixture into the prepared pie pan and bake for 45 to 50 minutes or until set.

Serve warm or cold.

Serves 5 to 6

# Kiwi Eggs

*We first tasted these in Rotorua, from one of the best self-taught Kiwi (New Zealander) chefs in the world. We change it a bit each time we make it. It serves as a great Balancing Protein when we want to include some elegant Comfort Food dessert in our Big Balanced Breakfast and need a bit of balance.*

1 tablespoon olive oil + additional if needed

2 teaspoons chopped scallions

4 hard-cooked eggs, peeled

2 patties low-fat turkey sausage, fully cooked, crumbled

⅛ teaspoon dried basil

Dash of ground black pepper

Dash of salt

½ green pepper, seeds removed, washed and dried

Heat the olive oil in a small saucepan over medium heat. Add the scallions and cook, stirring constantly, until they caramelize, 3 to 4 minutes. Remove from the heat and set aside.

Split the eggs in half, and place the whites on a serving plate and the yolks in a small bowl. Add the turkey sausage, basil, black pepper, and salt to the yolks and mix well. Add the scallions and thin with the pan drippings until the mixture becomes a thick paste. If necessary, add a little bit more olive oil to achieve the correct texture.

Fill the egg white halves with the mixture. Put the remaining mixture in the green pepper half.

Serve the eggs and green pepper immediately, or chill first and split the green pepper half into two equal portions.

Serves 2

# Hot and Spicy Turkey Sausage

*This sausage is high in tryptophan to balance serotonin in your brain and spicy hot to reduce cortisol levels. It's really good for breakfast, lunch, dinner, or in between with a dollop of prepared mustard and some crisp green pepper slices.*

2 pounds ground turkey

3 teaspoons crushed garlic

1 tablespoon soy sauce

2 teaspoons finely chopped fresh chile pepper, any variety (or to taste)

1 tablespoon dried sage

½ teaspoon ground black pepper

½ teaspoon dried basil

½ teaspoon nutmeg

½ teaspoon ground cloves

¼ cup olive oil

Combine the turkey, garlic, soy sauce, chile pepper, sage, black pepper, basil, nutmeg, and cloves in a large bowl, mixing well. Divide the mixture into 12 equal portions and shape each into a patty about 3½" in diameter.

Warm the oil in a large frying pan over medium heat. When the oil is hot, brown the patties on both sides for approximately 4 minutes on each side (making certain that they are cooked through).

Serve warm.

*Note: These patties freeze well for future use as a snack or as a delicious addition to other recipes.*

Makes 12

## SNACKS AND APPETIZERS

# Cracklin' Chicken

*Scientists have repeatedly documented the power of protein to satisfy. Chewing, as well, has the ability to bring satisfaction. When you combine the two, you have an all-around winner.*

*Our refrigerator and freezer are always stocked with Cracklin' Chicken. It's the perfect snack, appetizer, and side dish for any meal. We freeze it in meal-size portions. Whenever we like, we heat up a serving or two in the microwave (on very low) for 2 minutes. Voilà! Instant treat!*

> 2 boneless, skinless chicken breasts, each split in half
>
> 4 tablespoons teriyaki sauce + additional to taste
>
> 2 teaspoons garlic powder (or 8 teaspoons fresh minced garlic)
>
> ½ cup olive oil
>
> Salt and ground black pepper

Fill a large pot halfway with water. Bring to a moderate boil over medium heat. Add the chicken, teriyaki sauce, and garlic. Cover and cook for 30 minutes, or until the chicken is cooked through.

Drain the chicken, place it in a dish, and refrigerate.

When cool, shred the chicken with your hands. It should be stringy.

Warm the olive oil in a large skillet over medium-high heat. Add the shredded chicken and teriyaki sauce to taste. Stir constantly for about 3 to 5 minutes, until the chicken turns crispy and brown but does not burn.

To drain the cooking oil, remove the chicken with a slotted spatula to paper towel–lined plates. In 5 minutes, transfer to clean serving plates. Add salt and pepper to taste.

Serve warm, cool, refrigerate, or freeze.

Serves 6 to 8 as snacks or side dishes

# Buffalo Chicken Drumettes

*We used to wait until we went to our favorite restaurant for these. Then we real-ized we could make them (and make them better) ourselves.*

**Classic Buffalo Sauce**
½ cup hot-pepper sauce
1½ teaspoons cornstarch
¼ cup butter

1 pound chicken drumettes (the fleshy, lean part
  of a chicken wing)
3 tablespoons olive oil

Whisk the hot-pepper sauce and cornstarch until smooth in a small saucepan. Add the butter and warm over medium heat until the butter is melted.

Cook and stir constantly for 3 to 5 minutes, until the sauce thickens. Divide the sauce between two bowls, one large bowl for use with raw chicken, one medium bowl for cooked chicken.

Preheat the oven to 375°F.

Rinse the chicken drumettes. Blot dry with paper towels.

Transfer the drumettes, a few at a time, to the large mixing bowl. Stir to ensure that each drumette is covered with sauce.

Transfer the drumettes to a baking sheet coated thickly with olive oil. Discard any sauce remaining in the bowl. Bake for 45 minutes.

Wash your hands well with hot water and soap.

When the drumettes are thoroughly cooked, brush each with unused sauce.

Transfer to a clean serving dish and serve with Creamy Mustard Dipping Sauce (opposite), if desired.

Serves 3 to 4

# Creamy Mustard Dipping Sauce

*Smooth but tangy, this is the perfect Balancing Food dip for Balancing Proteins as well as Balancing Vegetables.*

3 ounces cream cheese

¼ cup olive oil

1 tablespoon white vinegar

2 teaspoons finely minced garlic

½ teaspoon prepared mustard

Salt and ground black pepper

Cut the cream cheese into small chunks. Place a few chunks in a bowl and beat with an electric mixer at low speed until smooth. Add the remaining cream cheese chunks, one at a time, beating after each addition until smooth.

Add the oil gradually, beating well. Add the vinegar, beating until blended. Add the garlic, mustard, and salt and pepper to taste, and beat until fully blended.

Chill and enjoy as a dip or dressing. Perfect with Buffalo Chicken Drumettes.

Makes approximately 1 cup

# Sensational Spicy Pumpkin Seeds

*Perfect for the Anxious Eater, the crunchiness of this treat will satisfy a desire to chew and help lower cortisol and adrenaline levels. Capsaicin in the cayenne pepper will signal the body to release endorphins, chemicals in the brain that bring pleasure and reduce stress naturally.*

1¼ cups hot water

½ elephant or regular garlic clove, crushed

2 cups roasted, shelled pumpkin seeds

1½ tablespoons butter, melted

1 teaspoon cayenne pepper

½ teaspoon salt

Preheat the broiler.

Combine the hot water and garlic in a medium saucepan. Mix well. Bring to a simmer over medium heat, stirring constantly.

Add the pumpkin seeds and simmer for 5 minutes, uncovered.

Drain the water, dry the seeds in paper towels, and set aside.

Combine the melted butter, cayenne pepper, and salt in the cooled, empty saucepan. Add the pumpkin seeds and stir until well coated.

Spread the seeds on a baking sheet. Toast under the broiler for 1 minute at a time, checking every minute until the seeds are lightly browned.

Serve warm or cold, sprinkled over a salad or tossed with Balancing Vegetables.

Makes 2 cups

# Shrimp Caliente

*Capsaicin in the cayenne pepper can raise oxytocin levels, increase pleasure, and reduce stress all at the same time.*

6 tablespoons olive oil

6 scallions, chopped

1 garlic clove, minced

1 pound large raw shrimp, peeled

¼ teaspoon ground black pepper

½ teaspoon cayenne pepper

¼ teaspoon paprika

Warm the oil in a medium skillet over medium heat. Add the scallions and garlic and cook, stirring often to prevent sticking, until the scallions begin to caramelize and turn dark green-brown.

Add the shrimp and stir constantly for 6 to 7 minutes, until they turn pink and are cooked through.

Remove from the heat and add the black pepper, cayenne pepper, and paprika. Stir well.

Serve warm.

Serves 2 to 3

## *MAIN DISHES*

# Athenian Pork Roast

*Black pepper is rich in chromium. Both the chromium and the Balancing Protein in this recipe will help keep insulin spikes from getting the upper hand.*

2 cups pitted and chopped green olives

1 cup roasted pistachios

2 pounds pork roast tenderloin, rinsed and patted dry

3 large garlic cloves, slivered

3 tablespoons olive oil

2 tablespoons paprika

2 tablespoons coarsely ground black pepper

Place an oven rack in the middle of the oven. Preheat the oven to 350°F.

Combine the olives and pistachios in a medium bowl. Set aside.

Using a sharp knife, make two lengthwise parallel slices, about 1" deep, along the top of the roast. Fill the slices with the mixture of olives and pistachios.

With the tip of the knife, make small, evenly spaced, 1" slits over the top of the roast. Insert a garlic sliver into each. Slowly pour the oil over the roast and sprinkle with the paprika and pepper.

Place the pork on a roasting rack in a shallow roasting pan. Cover the bottom of the pan with water to catch drippings and keep them from burning. Bake for 1½ hours or until the roast is cooked through.

Allow to cool for 5 to 10 minutes. Slice sideways so that each slice has a portion of the olive and pistachio mixture, and transfer the meat to a serving dish.

Serves 4 to 6

# Tuna-Mushroom Melt

*These are the perfect appetizer, snack, or light meal. The creamy texture of this flavorful delight will help lower the ghrelin levels that can cause cravings. This dish is filled with lots of chromium to balance your insulin levels, so it will keep you satisfied longer.*

8 large stuffing mushrooms

1 can (5 ounces) tuna, drained (preferably packed in olive oil)

¼ cup chopped celery

2 ounces cream cheese

½ tablespoon heavy cream

Salt and ground black pepper

Paprika

Place an oven rack in the middle of the oven and preheat the oven to 350°F. Scoop out the entire stalk of each mushroom and discard. Clean the mushroom caps well.

Place the tuna and celery in a medium bowl. Mix well with a fork. Add the cream cheese and cream, and mix well to combine. Add salt and pepper to taste.

Spoon generous portions of the mixture into each inverted mushroom cap. Set the mushroom caps in a shallow, oiled baking pan. Bake for 12 minutes. Sprinkle with paprika.

Serve warm.

Makes 8

# Scallops Diavolo

*A special blend of flavors gives this dish a surprising, stand-up-and-take-notice taste. The scallops, which are rich in magnesium, help reverse the mineral-depleting effects of adrenaline and cortisol.*

1 pound raw sea scallops, rinsed
⅛ cup teriyaki sauce
⅛ cup sweet Marsala wine
4 tablespoons olive oil
8 sprigs fresh parsley
4 tablespoons Dijon mustard
Salt and ground black pepper
Cayenne pepper

Preheat the oven to 425°F. Place the scallops in a single layer in an oiled baking dish.

Combine the teriyaki sauce, wine, olive oil, parsley, and mustard in a blender; process until smooth. Add salt, black pepper, and cayenne pepper to taste. Pour the mixture over the scallops.

Bake for 5 minutes, then turn once and baste. Bake for 5 to 7 minutes more. Season with additional salt, black pepper, and cayenne pepper to taste.

Serve warm.

Serves 3

# Pepper Steak with Pine Nuts

*Protein satisfies. Nuts satisfy as well. This alternative to a take-out Chinese dinner will balance your hormones, and it won't leave you hungry in an hour.*

¼ cup olive oil

1 cup raw, shelled pine nuts

1 pound beef fillet, cut in 1"–2" strips

1 garlic clove, minced

6 scallions, including green tops, sliced

3 green peppers, seeded and sliced into medium strips

3 ribs celery, sliced

2 tablespoons teriyaki sauce

Salt and pepper

Warm the olive oil in a large skillet over medium heat. Add the pine nuts and stir constantly for about 2 to 3 minutes. When the pine nuts turn golden brown, quickly remove them with a slotted spoon to a separate dish. Set aside.

Add the beef and garlic to the skillet. Brown, uncovered, for 3 minutes. Remove the meat with a slotted spoon and set aside.

Add the scallions, green peppers, and celery to the skillet. Stir for 3 minutes. Return the meat to the pan, add the teriyaki sauce, and continue stirring and cooking, uncovered, for 10 minutes, until the meat is cooked through. Add the pine nuts and stir quickly. Season with salt and pepper to taste. Remove from the heat and transfer to a serving dish.

Serve warm.

Serves 3 to 4

# Luscious and Legal Lasagna

*Enjoy this satisfying dish anytime. Equal parts Balancing Protein and Balancing Vegetables and Salad. Pure pleasure—no pasta! The spinach helps replenish the minerals that high levels of hormones can strip from your body.*

3 tablespoons olive oil

1 pound lean ground beef

4 scallions, chopped

1/2 green pepper, diced

1/2 garlic clove, thinly sliced

1/2 tablespoon dried basil

8 ounces ricotta cheese

1 egg, beaten

Salt and ground black pepper

8 ounces spinach, steamed and squeezed dry

4 ounces mozzarella cheese, shredded

Preheat the oven to 325°F.

Heat the olive oil in a large skillet over medium heat. Add the beef and cook until browned. Remove the beef and set aside.

Add the scallions, green pepper, and garlic to the same skillet with the drippings. Cook, stirring frequently, until the vegetables soften and begin to brown.

Add the beef and basil to the vegetable mixture and stir thoroughly. Remove from the heat. Set aside.

Combine the ricotta and egg in a medium bowl. Add salt and pepper to taste.

Grease a standard-size loaf pan with olive oil. Spread half of the meat mixture in the bottom of the pan. Top with all of the ricotta mixture. Top with the spinach, then half of the mozzarella. Cover with the remaining meat mixture, then top with the remaining mozzarella.

Bake for about 40 minutes or until the cheese is bubbly and starting to brown. Serve warm.

Serves 3 to 4

# Succulent Salmon with Almonds

*Researchers have found that eating fish and almonds provides a highly effective way to balance leptin and ghrelin levels and enhance weight loss. We would add that it's not only effective, it's very tasty as well![1]*

¼ cup Marsala wine

¼ cup teriyaki sauce

½ cup olive oil

2 teaspoons crushed garlic

Juice from 2 lemons

Black pepper

3 salmon steaks (4 ounces each)

1 cup raw almonds, coarsely ground

Whisk the wine, teriyaki sauce, olive oil, garlic, lemon juice, and pepper to taste in a medium bowl until blended. Place the salmon in a loaf pan, add the wine mixture, and marinate in the refrigerator for 2 hours.

Place oven racks in the middle and top positions of the oven. Preheat the broiler. Remove the salmon from the marinade and place on a broiling rack. Discard the marinade.

Broil on the middle rack for 4 to 5 minutes or until the salmon barely begins to brown. Turn over carefully. Broil for an additional 3 minutes.

Top with the almonds. Return the salmon to the top rack of the oven and broil for 1 more minute or until the salmon begins to flake slightly and the almonds are light brown. (Watch carefully to be certain the fish is cooked through but the nuts do not burn.)

Serve warm.

Serves 3

---

[1] Check with your physician regarding current recommendations.

# Tangy Asian Pork Ribs

*These ribs are packed with protein to lower ghrelin and insulin levels and cut cravings. They're also packed with flavor to leave you totally satisfied.*

2 pounds pork spareribs, lean and boneless,
cut into 3" segments

Salt and white pepper

¼ tablespoon minced garlic

¼ cup teriyaki sauce

¼ cup sweet Marsala wine

½ teaspoon grated lemon zest or 1 teaspoon lemon juice

2 cups olive oil

Sprinkle the ribs very lightly with equal parts salt and pepper, and rub it in well.

Mix the garlic, teriyaki sauce, wine, and lemon zest or juice in a large bowl. Add the spareribs, toss to coat, and marinate in the refrigerator for several hours.

In a small, deep frying pan, deep-fryer, or wok, heat the olive oil (use enough oil to cover the ribs) over medium heat until it reaches 320°F. Deep-fry the spareribs in batches until the pork is cooked through. Drain in a wire sieve or colander.

Serve warm.

Serves 6

## VEGETABLES AND SALADS

# Smooth and Sensuous Spinach Dip

*If it wasn't already known that smooth and creamy dishes help balance oxytocin levels, this dip would prove it. Plus, it's high in magnesium, which helps reverse the mineral-depleting effects of cortisol and adrenaline. This is a perfect warm dip to make Balancing Vegetables taste good. Enjoy it as a special reward for just being you.*

1 **package (10 ounces) frozen chopped spinach, defrosted, squeezed, and drained**

3 **ounces American cheese**

¼ **cup sour cream**

¼ **teaspoon ground black pepper**

1 **teaspoon minced garlic (or ¼ teaspoon garlic powder)**

**Salt**

**Hot-pepper sauce**

Place an oven rack in the middle of the oven. Preheat the oven to 350°F.

Combine the spinach, cheese, sour cream, pepper, garlic or garlic powder, and salt and hot-pepper sauce to taste in a large bowl. Transfer to a standard-size ovenproof glass loaf pan or 1-quart nonmetal baking dish.

Bake, uncovered, for 30 minutes.

Remove and transfer to a serving dish or individual serving bowls.

Serve with a wide variety of raw, finger-size portions of cauliflower, broccoli, mushroom caps, celery, green beans, or any other Balancing Vegetables that strike your fancy.

Serves 4 to 5

# Crunchy Crabmeat Salad

*Enjoy four-way satisfaction in this delicious dish: olive oil, protein, nuts, and citrus (high in vitamin C). Best of all, it's simple and quick to make and tastes great!*

2 tablespoons olive oil

1 pound cooked crabmeat (not imitation), cut into 2" chunks

Juice of 1 lemon

2 teaspoons dried basil

3 scallions, sliced crosswise

1 cup slivered almonds

½ teaspoon dried tarragon

Salt and coarsely ground black pepper

Parsley

Heat the olive oil in a medium skillet over medium heat until warm. Carefully add the crabmeat (it sizzles and spits). Stir constantly for 2 minutes or until warmed through. Do not overcook.

Remove from the heat and add the lemon juice, basil, scallions, almonds, tarragon, and salt and pepper to taste. Garnish with parsley, if desired.

Serve warm or cold.

Serves 3 to 4

# Baby Bok Choy with Cashews

*Softened bok choy will provide the chewiness; the cashews will provide the crunch. Scientists have found that crunchy, chewy foods reduce cortisol. Bet those same scientists wish they'd treated their subjects, and themselves, to this delicious non-meat, nondairy, hormone-balancing meal, snack, or side dish.*

- 1 pound baby bok choy, rinsed
- 2 tablespoons olive oil
- 5 large scallions, chopped
- ½ elephant or 1 regular garlic clove, chopped
- ½ teaspoon sesame oil
- 1 teaspoon teriyaki sauce
- ½ cup chopped, roasted cashews

Place the bok choy on a cutting board. Remove the larger leaves by separating them from the base. Trim the base of the bok choy carefully to leave it holding the smaller leaves in place.

Warm the olive oil in a large pan over medium heat. Add the scallions. Cook, stirring frequently, for about 30 seconds. Add the garlic and cook for another 30 seconds. Add the bok choy. Turn it in the olive oil, scallion, and garlic mixture until it's coated on all sides. Add the sesame oil and teriyaki sauce and turn to coat.

Cover and cook over medium-low heat for 3 to 4 minutes or until wilted.

Uncover and stir for a few minutes longer until the bok choy is cooked but not too soft. Gently mix in the cashews, lifting the bok choy with tongs or two forks to avoid breaking it.

Serve warm.

Serves 3 to 4

# Chipotle Turkey Salad

*Turkey is rich in tryptophan and can help raise serotonin levels naturally. The result: a spicy dish that won't give you after-cravings. By the way, chicken works just as well. Contrary to popular belief, chicken contains more tryptophan than turkey.*

2½ cups cubed cooked turkey

1 cup mayonnaise

½ large green pepper, diced

2 scallions, sliced

1 chipotle pepper in adobo sauce, minced,
   or 2 tablespoons chipotle salsa

Garlic powder

Combine the turkey, mayonnaise, green pepper, scallions, and chipotle pepper or salsa in a large bowl. Stir until evenly combined and coated with mayonnaise. Season with garlic powder to taste.

Serve with celery sticks or wrap in lettuce leaves.

Serves 2

# Green Beans Amandine

*Rich in antioxidants, green beans help fight the effects of cortisol. The high fiber works well to keep ghrelin, insulin, and stress cravings low. Sesame seeds are rich in plant compounds known as phytosterols, which help keep cortisol levels down. Best of all, these beans are simply delicious.*

2 pounds fresh green beans

½ cup olive oil

2 tablespoons minced garlic

¼ cup sesame seeds

⅓ cup slivered, blanched almonds

Salt and pepper

Wash the beans and cut off the ends. Drain and set aside.

Pour the olive oil into a medium frying pan and place over medium heat. Add the garlic and cook, stirring constantly, until fragrant (about 2 minutes). Reduce the heat to low and add the sesame seeds. Cook, stirring, until the sesame seeds just begin to toast. Add the almonds. Raise the heat to medium and stir until the first almond sliver begins to brown. Immediately add the green beans and stir constantly for about 3 minutes. Remove from the heat and add salt and pepper to taste. The beans should still be crisp.

Serve warm. Can be sprinkled with teriyaki sauce, lemon juice, or wine vinegar.

Serves 4

# COMFORT FOOD RECIPES
## BREAKFASTS
# Unforgettable French Toast

*Big Balanced Breakfast pleasure. Add breakfast meat, then sit back and enjoy!*

3 **eggs**

2 **tablespoons honey**

4 **tablespoons cream (light or heavy)**

4 **slices white bread**

4 **tablespoons butter + extra for frying, if needed**

1 **banana, sliced**

**Confectioners' sugar and cinnamon (optional)**

Whisk together the eggs, honey, and cream in a large bowl. Transfer 2 slices of bread to the mixture, making certain both slices are immersed. Set aside.

Melt the butter in a medium skillet over medium heat. Add the banana slices and cook, stirring frequently, until warmed and covered in melted butter (about 1 minute). Remove and set aside.

Gently transfer the egg-soaked bread to the skillet and cook, adding additional butter as necessary to prevent sticking.

As the first 2 slices cook, immerse the second 2 slices of bread in the remaining egg mixture and set aside.

When the first 2 slices of bread are browned on the bottom, use a spatula to carefully turn and brown them on the other side. When cooked through, transfer to a serving plate.

Cook the remaining 2 slices of bread.

Meanwhile, top the French toast on the serving plate with the banana slices. Top with the remaining French toast when it's cooked through. If desired, lightly sprinkle with confectioners' sugar and cinnamon. Serve warm and delicious.

Serves 2

# Cream-of-Wheat Pancakes

*What a way to get your serving of hot cereal! This dish includes a nice portion of Balancing Protein even though it tastes like it's all Comfort Food.*

1¼ cups all-purpose flour

⅓ cup instant cream of wheat

⅓ cup sugar

1 teaspoon baking soda

1 teaspoon baking powder

½ teaspoon salt

¼ cup milk

½ cup sour cream

¼ cup canola oil

1 egg

1 teaspoon vanilla extract

6 tablespoons butter

Mix the flour, cream of wheat, sugar, baking soda, baking powder, and salt in a large bowl and set aside.

Whisk together the milk, sour cream, canola oil, egg, and vanilla in a medium bowl.

Make a well in the center of the dry ingredients. Pour in the wet ingredients and blend with a fork until the liquid is well distributed. Do not overmix.

Heat a large skillet over medium heat. In the skillet, melt 1 tablespoon butter, or more as needed.

Pour approximately one-sixth of the batter onto the skillet and cook until bubbles appear on the surface. Flip with a spatula and cook until browned on the other side. Repeat until all of the batter is used.

Finished pancakes may be kept warm on the ovenproof plate in the oven (approximately 250°F), while remaining pancakes are cooked.

Serve warm.

Makes 6

# Old-Fashioned Sour Cream Biscuits

*Pure Comfort Food. These biscuits are the perfect complement to a hearty, protein-rich main dish.*

½ cup sour cream

¼ cup milk

1½ tablespoons canola or corn oil

1 cup all-purpose flour

1 cup pastry flour

1 tablespoon sugar

1½ teaspoons baking powder

½ teaspoon baking soda

½ teaspoon salt

1½ tablespoons cold butter, sliced

1 tablespoon milk

Preheat the oven to 425°F. Coat a baking sheet with canola or corn oil cooking spray.

Combine the sour cream and milk in a small bowl. Add the oil, mix, and set aside.

Whisk together the flours, sugar, baking powder, baking soda, and salt in a large bowl. Using your fingertips or 2 knives in a scissors fashion, cut the butter into the dry ingredients until crumbly. Make a small well in the center of the mixture and slowly pour in the sour cream mixture, stirring with a fork until just combined and forming a dough.

Transfer the dough to a floured surface and sprinkle the top lightly with flour. Gently knead the dough no more than 7 or 8 times. Pat or roll out to ¾" thickness. Cut into 2" rounds and transfer to the prepared baking sheet. Brush the tops with the milk.

Bake for 11 to 15 minutes, until golden brown. Transfer to a wire rack and allow to cool slightly before serving.

Makes 10

# Powerhouse Pancakes

*Don't judge a pancake by its ingredients! This one contains cottage cheese, but you'd never know it. We wouldn't have put it in the Comfort Foods recipe section if it wasn't that good!*

2 eggs, separated

1 cup small-curd cottage cheese

½ cup all-purpose flour

Salt

Dash of cinnamon (optional)

⅛ teaspoon cream of tartar

1 tablespoon canola oil

**Topping (Optional):**
2–3 tablespoons sour cream sweetened with
    1 teaspoon sugar

Preserves of choice

Combine the egg yolks, cottage cheese, flour, salt to taste, and cinnamon, if desired, in a medium bowl. Set aside.

Beat the egg whites and cream of tartar in a separate bowl until stiff but not dry. Fold into the cottage cheese mixture. Set aside.

Spray a large skillet or square griddle with canola oil cooking spray or grease it with butter or canola oil and warm it over medium heat. Drop the batter by large spoonfuls onto the hot surface. Fry the pancakes until bubbles appear around the edges and they are golden brown on one side; turn and brown the other sides.

Serve at once, either plain, with sour cream topping, or topped with a spoonful or two of preserves.

Makes 4 pancakes (4")

## *MAIN DISHES*

# Succulent Sweet-and-Sour Pork

*Chinese food at your fingertips without the glutamates. Add Balancing Vegetables and Salad and you're ready to go.*

1 can (15¼ ounces) pineapple chunks

1 pound boneless pork loin

2 tablespoons olive oil + additional if needed

1 medium green or red pepper, cut into 1" chunks

1 medium onion, minced

¼ cup brown sugar

¼ cup white vinegar

2 tablespoons cornstarch

2 tablespoons teriyaki sauce

Hot cooked rice (optional)

Drain the pineapple, reserving the juice. Set aside.

Cut the pork loin across the grain into 2½" cubes. Heat a wok or large skillet over high heat and add the oil. Add the pepper and onion and stir-fry for 2 to 3 minutes or until the pepper is crisp but tender. Remove the pepper and onion and set aside. Add more oil as needed to the wok or skillet. Add half the pork and stir-fry until browned. Remove and set aside. Stir-fry the remaining pork. Reduce the heat to low. Return all of the pork to the wok or skillet to keep warm, stirring occasionally.

Combine the pineapple juice, brown sugar, vinegar, cornstarch, and teriyaki sauce in a small saucepan. Bring to a boil. Cook for 1 minute or until thickened, stirring constantly. Remove from the heat and set aside.

Return the pepper and onion to the wok or skillet and mix with the pork. Stir in the pineapple and thickened pineapple juice mixture. Increase the heat to medium. Cook and stir until heated through.

If served with rice, include some additional Balancing Protein (with Balancing Vegetables and Salad, if appropriate) for balance.

Serves 4

# Fried Chicken with a Tangy Twist

*A new variation on an old-time favorite. It's a Comfort Food recipe that is so rich in protein it will help balance any meal that includes a very rich dessert.*

½ cup seasoned dry bread crumbs

1 teaspoon ground black pepper

1 teaspoon salt

1 teaspoon paprika

2 teaspoons garlic powder

1 cup flour

½ cup milk

1 egg

1 cup olive oil

4 boneless, skinless chicken breast halves, pounded thin

2 lemons, split, seeds removed

Combine the bread crumbs, pepper, salt, paprika, garlic powder, and flour in a shallow dish. Set aside.

Whisk the milk and egg in a medium bowl. Set aside.

Heat the oil over medium-low heat or in an electric skillet set to 350°F.

Dip the chicken into the milk mixture, then dredge in the flour mixture until evenly coated.

Fry the chicken in the hot oil for about 5 to 6 minutes per side, or until it's cooked through and the juices run clear.

Remove from the oil with a slotted spatula and place on a serving plate. Squeeze the juice from half a lemon over each chicken breast. Serve warm or as a delicious leftover.

Serves 4

# Block Island Beef Stew

*Beef stew, thy name is Comfort Food!*

> ¼ cup olive oil
>
> 2 pounds stew beef, cut into 1" pieces
>
> 2 large garlic cloves, minced
>
> 8 cups beef stock or canned beef broth (no MSG added)
>
> 2 tablespoons tomato paste
>
> 3 tablespoons sugar
>
> 1 tablespoon Worcestershire sauce
>
> 2 bay leaves
>
> 1 tablespoon dried thyme
>
> 5 tablespoons teriyaki sauce
>
> 3 tablespoons Marsala wine
>
> 2 tablespoons butter
>
> 1 pound potatoes, washed, peeled, and cut into ½" chunks
>
> 1 large onion, chopped
>
> 5 carrots, washed, peeled, and cut into thick slices

Warm the oil in a large pot over medium-high heat. Add the beef and cook, stirring, until browned on all sides (about 7 minutes). Add the garlic and cook, stirring, for 2 minutes. Add the beef stock or broth, tomato paste, sugar, Worcestershire, bay leaves, thyme, teriyaki sauce, and wine. Stir well. Bring the mixture to a boil. Reduce heat to medium-low, cover, and simmer for 1 hour, stirring occasionally.

Meanwhile, melt the butter in a medium skillet over medium heat. Add the potatoes, onion, and carrots. Cook, stirring frequently, until golden, about 15 minutes. Add the vegetables to the beef stew.

Simmer, uncovered, until the beef is cooked through and both the beef and vegetables are tender, about 40 to 50 minutes more. Remove and discard the bay leaves. Spoon off any fat that may have settled on top.

Serve warm with Old-Fashioned Sour Cream Biscuits (see page 278).

Serves 5 to 6

# Simply Chili

*We make a huge soup pot of this hearty meal, package it in freezer bags, and enjoy it for several weeks whenever we like. Packed with satisfying protein, it's already balanced with half Balancing Protein and half Comfort Food.*

¼ cup olive oil

3 pounds lean ground beef

1 medium onion, chopped

2 garlic cloves, crushed

1 can (28 ounces) crushed tomatoes

8 ounces kidney beans, rinsed and drained

8 ounces chickpeas, rinsed and drained

2 tablespoons chili powder, or to taste

Warm the olive oil in a large skillet over medium heat. Add the ground beef, onion, and garlic, and cook, stirring frequently, until the beef is browned. Drain and discard the oil. Add the tomatoes, kidney beans, and chickpeas. Stir well. Bring to a simmer, stirring often. Reduce the heat to low, cover, and cook for 30 minutes, stirring often. Add the chili powder in ½-tablespoon increments, stirring and tasting after each addition. Simmer uncovered for 30 minutes longer, stirring occasionally. Serve warm.

If you serve with the Old-Fashioned Sour Cream Biscuits (page 278), add a dollop of sour cream and some Balancing Vegetables and Salad for a perfect Alternative Meal.

Serves 8

## DESSERTS

# Chocolate Silk

*A cross between chocolate pudding and a crustless chocolate cheesecake; save this one for a special treat. Balance this dessert with a good portion of Balancing Foods, and you have an unforgettable Big Balanced Breakfast or Alternative Meal. Amazingly satisfying!*

> 8 ounces cream cheese
> 8 ounces sour cream
> 2 eggs
> $\frac{1}{2}$ cup sugar
> $\frac{1}{2}$ cup cocoa

Preheat the oven to 350°F.

Cut the cream cheese into 1" squares. Set aside.

Place the sour cream in the bowl of an electric mixer. Begin mixing at the lowest speed. While mixing, immediately add the eggs, one at a time. Mix in the sugar, then one or two cream cheese cubes at a time until all are thoroughly blended. Add the cocoa slowly, 1 heaping tablespoon at a time. Mix well at low speed.

Spoon into four 12-ounce ovenproof bowls. Bake for 20 minutes. Serve warm or cool.

Makes 4 servings

*Variation: Break 2 bars of semisweet chocolate (4 ounces each) into large bite-size pieces. Mix in before baking.*

# Quick-and-Easy Coffee Cake

*We haven't bothered to sift the ingredients. And, in general, it doesn't seem to make a difference. This just-sweet-enough dessert is the perfect finish for a Big Balanced Breakfast or an Alternative Meal lunch or dinner. Freeze extra wedges and heat in the microwave for an instant and satisfying dessert.*

1¾ cups flour

2 teaspoons baking powder

½ teaspoon salt

½ cup sugar

6 tablespoons cold butter, sliced

1 egg, beaten

½ cup milk

1½ tablespoons butter, melted

**Topping**

3 tablespoons flour

¾ teaspoon ground cinnamon

¾ cup sugar

Preheat the oven to 400°F. Grease a 9" layer pan with canola oil cooking spray or a tablespoon of butter.

Combine the flour, baking powder, salt, and sugar in a medium bowl. Mix with a fork. Cut the butter into the dry ingredients with a fork or pastry blender. Set aside.

Combine the egg and milk in a small bowl. Beat well with a fork. Add to the flour mixture. Stir until the mixture is smooth. Spoon into the prepared pan, spreading evenly. Brush the top of the dough with the melted butter.

For the topping, combine the flour, cinnamon, and sugar in a small bowl. Spoon over the cake. Spread with a fork to cover the dough evenly.

Bake for 25 to 35 minutes or until a butter knife inserted into the center comes out clean. Cut in wedges and serve warm.

Serves 6

# Index

## A

activities. *See* hormone balancing activities or adventures
addiction. *See* carbohydrate addiction
adrenal fatigue, 38–39
adrenaline
  adrenaline resistance, 103
  adventure for increasing, 188–89
  bedtime decline of, 96
  breathing to balance, 187
  capsaicin for increasing, 188
  cortisol increasing, 64, 72
  dopamine as building-block for, 74
  dopamine competing with, 74–75
  fat-making mode maintained by, 87
  foods increasing, 192
  functions of, 31
  high, health problems from, 187
  increase with low oxytocin, 92
  insulin sensitivity reduced by, 66, 187
  Masters of Metabolism summoned by, 4
  meditation for reducing, 191–92
  mineral-depleting effects of, 266, 271
  morning levels of, 124
  Night-Eating Syndrome and, 96–97
  oxytocin competing with, 64–65
  oxytocin increase with low, 95, 96
  oxytocin reduced by, 64
  oxytocin reducing, 65, 69, 184–85, 205
  planning for pleasure to increase, 189–90
  pleasurable rushes from, 73
  prizefighter exercise to increase, 187
  self-perpetuating cycle of, 74
  Sensational Spicy Pumpkin Seeds for reducing, 262
  signs of high levels of, 56
  social situations affected by, 65
  Stress-Eating Patterns and
    Anxiety-Induced Stress-Eaters, 86, 87, 205
    Exhaustion-Induced Stress-Eaters, 103
    Frustration-Induced Stress-Eaters, 64, 65–66, 183–84
    Guilt-Induced Stress-Eaters, 95, 96
    Quicky Stress-Eaters, 105, 217
    Secret Stress-Eaters, 78, 194, 196
    Self-Sacrificing Stress-Eaters, 72–75, 191–93
    Social Stress-Eaters, 69–70, 186–90
    Task-Avoiding Stress-Eaters, 92, 208
  in Stress-Eating Rebound, 35
  stress-hunger from, 73–74
  in Stress-Resistors, 31
  in Stress-Responders, 35
  sugar substitutes increasing, 192, 193
adrenaline resistance, 103
adventures. *See* hormone balancing activities or adventures
aging, stress-eating increase with, 45
alcoholic drinks, 137, 252
almonds
  in Crunchy Crabmeat Salad, 272
  in Green Beans Amandine, 275
  Succulent Salmon with Almonds, 269
Alternative Meal. *See also* Step #1: Cutting Cravings
  alcoholic drinks with, 137
  Balancing Vegetables and Salad in, 143, 154
  Big Balanced Breakfast compared to, 143
  Big Balanced Breakfast replaced by, 116, 123, 132, 133, 141
  carbo drift with, 215
  defined, 116, 195, 215
  diet drinks with, 193
  guidelines for, 142–43
  if benefits are lacking with, 143
  non–Big Balanced Breakfast continued with, 142, 143
  recipes recommended for
    Chocolate Silk, 284
    Crustless Mushroom Quiche, 256